ACID REFLUX DIET

Complete Guide to Prevent, Treat Gerd and Acid Reflux With
Natural Remedies

(The Ultimate Combo to Get Rid of Acid Reflux)

Donald Malec

Published by Alex Howard

© **Donald Malec**

All Rights Reserved

Acid Reflux Diet: Complete Guide to Prevent, Treat Gerd and Acid Reflux With Natural Remedies (The Ultimate Combo to Get Rid of Acid Reflux)

ISBN 978-1-77485-002-2

Legal & Disclaimer

The information contained in this book is not designed to replace or take the place of any form of medicine or professional medical advice. The information in this book has been provided for educational and entertainment purposes only.

Table of contents

Part 1

CHAPTER 1: WHAT IS ACID REFLUX?

Acid reflux disease has just come into the media spotlight recently. This is because of the development of different medications and treatments for acid reflux. In other words, because, drug companies can make some money from finding a cure for acid reflux, there seems to be a sudden outbreak of acid reflux disease.

Acid reflux disease explained in the easiest way possible is when you keep vomiting a little bit at a time. This not only does it put a terrible taste in your mouth, but it is also very uncomfortable.

Basically, you have stomach acid constantly being in your esophagus going up or going back down. Stomach acid is not meant to be in your esophagus for long periods of time and the acid eventually can greatly damage your esophagus which makes eating very difficult. You can also possibly get cancer of the esophagus, which is the worst possible scenario.

There are many causes for acid reflux and an explanation is needed on why so much stomach acid is in your esophagus and not in your stomach. Most of the time it is because of your lifestyle decisions that a person makes that cause acid reflux disease. If you are not exercising, not eating healthy or continue to smoke "cancer sticks" and drink alcohol you are a prime candidate for acid reflux disease.

Pregnancy can also cause acid reflux because the baby is pressing on your stomach. But at least you know this kind of acid reflux will eventually go away in 9 months or sooner. Unfortunately, the other kinds of acid reflux does not go away this easily and need to be addressed by a doctor. If you have heartburn or think you might have acid reflux, explained or unexplained, go see your doctor. The doctor can determine what kind of acid reflux you have and what the probable cause is and help get you the best treatment that you need.

Acid Reflux is very similar to heartburn, but acid reflux is a lot more uncomfortable than heartburn and definitely leads to a lot more potential health problem.

Aquick way to find out if "it's just heartburn" is to take an over the counter heartburn relief medication. If you do not feel better from the medication and you can barely get a good night's sleep because of the acid burning in your throat you probably do have acid reflux disease.

Since acid reflux can now be explained there are a number of new medications that can help alleviate the problem. There are a lot of new prescription medications which many acid reflux sufferers are happy with and some that are not so pleased with.

Other alternatives include changing your sleeping position with special foam wedges and pillows to keep your body slightly inclined. This way the acid stays within its regular area of the stomach.

If you can learn some techniques for handling stress, especially if you get an upset stomach whenever you are upset or under pressure will help cure your acid reflux. Finally, watching what you eat and eating healthier can really go a long way in curing your acid reflux condition.

CHAPTER 2: ACID REFLUX; THE CAUSE, AND THE SYMPTOMS

Not sure what that burning in your chest means? Two words that make your day a living nightmare, "Acid Reflux"! You have put up with the misery for maybe months and possibly years and it's time to do something about it! Acid Reflux or GERD (also called heartburn) affects millions of people each day and might be affecting you! The first step of action is to educate yourself on acid reflux and discover how you might naturally treat your heartburn.

THE CAUSE OF ACID REFLUX

There are numerous causes of Acid Reflux but knowing they could possibly allow you to find your problem. It might be a small habit you need to change or a drastic lifestyle makeover. Whatever the cause, it is necessary for you to take it seriously and make the adjustmentquickly. The following is a list of causes for Acid Reflux:

1. Too much caffeine (coffee, tea, soda and chocolate) can cause Acid Reflux.

2. Consumption of alcohol (wine or beer) can cause Acid Reflux.

3. Smoking cigarettes can cause Acid Reflux.

4. Eating large meals can cause Acid Reflux.

5. Eating 2-3 hours before bedtime can cause Acid Reflux.

6. High-fat foods (especially fried foods) can cause Acid Reflux.

7. Foods containing tomatoes cause Acid Reflux.

8. Fruits and fruit juices cause Acid Reflux.

9. Tight fitting clothes around midsection can cause Acid Reflux.

THE SYMPTOMS OF ACID REFLUX

At its most basic, Gastroesophageal reflux disease (GERD), or acid reflux, is a condition where the stomach backs up (refluxes) and the acid within returns into the esophagus. If you are wondering if you suffer from acid reflux, the following are typical symptoms of Acid Reflux.

1. Heartburn (burning sensation ranging from the upper stomach to lower chest)

2. Regurgitation (food brought back up into the mouth)

3. Slight to Harsh Chest Pains

4. Difficulty in swallowing

5. Hoarseness in speaking

6. Dental erosion from stomach acids in mouth and throat

7. Asthma and/or a cough

CHAPTER 3: THE GERD DIET

Acid reflux or Gastroesophageal Reflux disease (GERD) is a simple, yet sometimes a disease that can be both painful and chronic. The GERD diet is a part of a total treatment plan that includes both lifestyle changes and medication as well as dietary changes.

A diet plan is necessary to both reducing pain and allows healing in the affected areas of the esophagus. The changes in this specific diet include eating less and eating foods that are tolerated and thus eliminate the painful symptoms of acid reflux.

The GERD diet is only one part of an acid reflux treatment plan. A diet is used to prevent advancement of the disease and allow for healing in the affected organs. The diet consists of foods that are mild and do not cause a relaxation of pressure in the stomach, thereby opening the lower esophageal sphincter (LES).

The meals are lighter and eating before bedtime is eliminated. These are done in order to prevent acid reflux symptoms during the night. Before beginning a GERD diet plan you keep a food diary listing foods that are eaten, how much and all symptoms that are felt in addition to the severity of pain. This is used to determine what foods are causing the symptoms and what foods seem to help.

Chewing gum has been found to promote the continual production of saliva. This saliva has a high PH level and it is possible that it can promote a natural antacid effect upon the LES. Therefore, gum chewing on the GERD diet is encouraged whenever possible.

The diet, as stated above, makes use of the completed food diary and eliminates all foods that have previously caused acid reflux. In addition, with the GERD diet, it is recommended that all meals are lighter, especially in the evening hours before bedtime. This helps prevent nighttime occurrences.

Milk, previously thought by some to prevent acid reflux, has been shown to actually cause it when taken before bed. So drinking of milk before bed is prohibited. Alcohol is also prohibited as it has been known to cause acid reflux.

However, coffee, which previously had been automatically eliminated on the GERD diet is now allowed as tolerated, as it has been shown that not everyone is sensitive to coffee.

On the GERD diet other foods, also previously prohibited such as peppermint, spearmint, and chocolate, as well as hot and spicy foods, are also allowed as tolerated.

This is because the theory that milk cures ulcers and acid reflux and hot, spicy foods aggravate, it has been found to be somewhat of a myth. The GERD diet is one way you can get relief from your heartburn.

It is also an important aspect of acid reflux treatment and it is used to prevent severe complications of your GERD. So, be sure to follow your doctor or nutritionist's advice if they put you on a GERD diet.

CHAPTER 4: SIMPLE STEPS TO HELP AGAINST GERD - ACID REFLUX DISEASE

There are many people who are being diagnosed with GERD. As strange as this may sound, GERD is commonly known as Acid Reflux Disease. I have a nephew who complained of nausea in the morning, stomach aches, and a sore throat.

After going to the doctor, he was diagnosed with gastroesophageal reflux disease, (GERD). This is a medical condition where the liquids from the stomach go back up into the esophagus.

The liquid contains stomach acids and can inflame and damage the lining of the esophagus. Fortunately, treatment is available for GERD. By changing your diet, taking the right types of medicines and modifying your sleeping habits, your GERD symptoms could diminish.

1. DIET

Certain foods can promote GERD. They reduce the amount of pressure in the lower esophageal muscle and cause the "reflux" to occur. Avoiding the following foods will help Chocolate, peppermint, alcohol, Fatty Foods, caffeinated drinks and even smoking.

At meal time, try eating smaller meals earlier in the evening. The smaller meals will help keep the acids from going up the esophagus. By eating earlier, your stomach will have had a chance to fully digest your food.

Chewing gum can help reduce acid in the esophagus by increasing saliva production. Once swallowed, the saliva helps neutralizes acid in the esophagus.

2. TAKING THE RIGHT MEDICINES

Don't take plain old antacid tablets. These will only help for a very short time. There are two types of medicines on the market today specifically designed to help the symptoms of GERD. The first medicine developed specifically for the treatment of acid-related disorders was Tagamet. This product and others like it (Zantac, Axid & Pepcid) were designed to neutralize acids in the stomach.

Your stomach will continue to naturally produce acid, but these products will counteract that acid by neutralizing it. This type of medicine is best used 1/2 hour before a meal so it can get to work and be ready for the food digestion process.

These same medicines can be taken just before bed to help reduce the number of harmful acids being produced. Newer medicines have been created that work differently than these acid neutralizers just mentioned. Known as Proton Pump Inhibitors (PPI), these drugs actually block the production of antacids into the stomach.

Since the acid production is turned off, it will help prevent acid from going up the esophagus and promote healing from the burning and inflammation that is caused by Acid Reflux. Brands like Prilosec, Nexium, Protonix, and Prevacid are all PPI-type drugs and usually involve a doctor's script.

3. SLEEPING HABITS

Believe it or not, the way you sleep can promote GERD. Laying flat on your back allows the stomach acids to easily evacuate up into your esophagus. Elevate your bed where your head is positioned. Using a simple bed pillow to elevate your head won't help.

You need to elevate your upper body too. There are special wedge pillows available that are designed to do just this. For about 25 - 30 dollars you can sleep better at night. As always, consult your doctor about your health. Do not self-diagnose and always read the directions, warnings, and instructions on any medication you take.

The symptoms you are experiencing could be a more serious problem not related to GERD. Having said that, the simple changes to your diet, sleeping habits and the right medicines could significantly help your Acid Reflux Disease. Seek help and feel better.

CHAPTER 5: ACID REFLUX RECIPES

When acid reflux becomes a regular part of life, the sufferer is commonly advised to change his or her diet. Try to avoid citrus, Try to avoid acids. See if the changes make it better. So you try. You experiment. And all the time, you're wishing there were acid reflux cure recipes. You finally go looking for such, and you find that there are cookbooks that focus on eating to avoid acid reflux.

The trouble is that neither you nor your doctor can say for sure that your current diet is the problem. You hate to put out money for an acid reflux cookbook only to learn that your acid reflux stems from another cause.

You'd like to find someone that inserts one little word in the phrase acid reflux cure recipes.

A. ACID REFLUX FREE CURE RECIPES

If you could just find acid reflux free cure recipes, you would try them. If it turned out that they did help, you wouldn't mind investing in one or two good acid reflux recipe cookbooks.

Acid reflux free cure recipes have three things in common.

1. They eliminate or reduce portions of those foods that are typically difficult to digest.

2. They include or increase portions of those foods that are known to aid in digestion.

3. They are FREE!

Orange juice, for example, is acidic. Many people claim that it increases acid reflux. So replace breakfast orange juice with a ripe banana, which is easy to digest. Or opt for an apple. Brownies and donuts are considered foods to be avoided by acid reflux sufferers.

They tend to sit, undigested, in the stomach. Choose an easily digested dessert such as a fat-free cookie or jelly beans.

ACID REFLUX RECIPE IDEAS

Here is a handful of ideas for acid reflux recipes.

1. Waldorf salad, made with ripe, healthy apples, nuts, and raisins, is a good acid reflux cure recipe. Use any traditional Waldorf salad recipe, but substitute low-fat mayonnaise and sour cream. You will have a great-tasting salad that contains no recognized acid reflux trigger foods.

2. Beef stew is another great acid reflux cure recipe. Use any beef stew recipe you like, omitting the onions. Cut the fat from the beef. If the stew seems to trigger acid reflux, eat a smaller portion next time.

3. Gingerbread is a marvelous dessert for acid reflux sufferers. Find a recipe that uses canned pumpkin and wheat germ. Make it with unsweetened applesauce and low-fat buttermilk. Then resist the temptation to mound whipped cream on top of it! Try a low-fat imitation whip instead.

4. Roast turkey breast is a good main course. Cranberries should be fine with it. Serve the potato, baked instead of mashed.

5. Lowly meatloaf is thought to have no specific acid reflux triggers.

6. Spaghetti may cause acid reflux in some. You can reduce the possibilities by beginning with acid-free tomato sauce. Omit garlic and onion from your sauce, and try using more basil and less oregano. There are a number of Italian spices that are great in spaghetti sauce. Try fennel with basil.

7. Cheesecake, too, can be an acid reflux cure recipe. Make it with reduced fat or no-fat cheeses. Use egg whites and/or egg substitute. While trying your acid reflux free cure recipes, learn what the actual cause of acid reflux is. You may be surprised to know that it is a muscular problem. There may be things you can do other than altering your diet.

Also for better understanding;

1. Consume food that is rich in complex carbohydrates

Foods that are good for an acid reflux diet are foods that contain complex carbohydrates. Foods such as bread, pasta, and rice tend to absorb the acid and prevent it from backing up into the esophagus. Since these foods tend to put on weight, it is better to eat smaller portions of them. If you drink milk, switch to a milk that is lower in fat.

2. Stick to non-carbonated drinks

Switch to drinks without carbonation. Decaf tea or coffee is a good choice but water is better. There are many flavored glasses of water that are quite good and good for you. Herbal tea is another good choice. You can experiment with the foods you eat to determine which foods cause you the most trouble. Everybody reacts to foods differently. By controlling your portions and eating high acid foods in moderation, you should be able to stick to an acid reflux diet without a lot of difficulties.

3. Use a nutritious meat

There are some excellent meats to include in this diet that is nutritious and delicious. Extra lean ground beef, steak, and chicken are usually great for the main course when on the best diet for acid reflux. Most fish is also very nutritious and safe for those with acid reflux. All of these are acceptable in the best diet for acid reflux, but these should not be cooked with a lot of greases. Those who want to avoid the symptoms of acid reflux might want to grill or broil the dishes.

4. Use wheat based food items

Most bread, cereal and graham crackers should not produce the symptoms of acid reflux. Cornbread and pretzels are good additions to the best diet fiber acid reflux. The best diet for acid reflux will eliminate some desserts, but other desserts should be fine for those with this condition.

5. Use cheese

Cheese often makes a good dessert, and there are some cheeses that will be an important part of the best diet for acid reflux. Fat-free cookies are usually fine for those with acid reflux. People with acid reflux should avoid rich, creamy cakes and most ice creams.

6. Use ginger

Gingers have some healingqualities, and those with acid reflux might try adding ginger to some of their food and beverages. Fresh ginger is available in the grocery stores, and this can be ground up and added to meals. Some dishes call for this in the recipe, but it can be added to other dishes. Ginger can also be added to tea. There are some cuisines that include ginger in many dishes such as Chinese cuisine. Those with acid reflux might patronize the Chinese restaurants and look for those dishes with ginger.

7. Drink tea

People with acid reflux should try to add green tea to their diet as this beverage is known to help the body digest other food and beverages. Herbal teas contain substances such as chamomile and licorice root provide a repair mechanism for the stomach so those with acid reflux should consume these teas if possible.

People with acid reflux should try to drink plenty of water, which will help the body excrete the excess acid more efficiently.

CHAPTER 6: GUIDELINES ON PROPER ACID REFLUX DIETS AND FOOD TO AVOID

Before taking medication, most doctors will advise that the person with acid reflux disease make some changes to his/her diet, i.e. have a proper acid reflux diet plan. It is an easy and useful change that one can make. A proper diet for acid reflux could make a huge difference to the health and comfort of many people.

With a proper diet for acid reflux, it could remove all of the symptoms attributed to this condition and provide for a more undisturbed sleep. An effective and proper acid reflux diet plan includes knowing what food to avoid, what food to consume and good eating habits.

In this book, we shall go through some important guidelines that you can take away.

1. Avoid spicy food

Stay away from spicy foods. Even foods you don't think taste spiciness can play a big role in creating acid reflux, so knowing what's in your food and knowing to stay away from food with spices in them is a great way to naturally remedy acid reflux. This isn't to say you are limited to nothing but bland foods now, it just means be as liberal as possible when eating spices that can irritate your stomach to the point of being in pain.

21

2. Cut down on large meals

A recommended choice of acid reflux diet plan has always included eating several small meals every day instead of three large meals as what most people do. This is a good eating habit for everyone, even if you don't experience from acid reflux disease. This is to let the stomach to have sufficient capacity for proper digestion.

3. Avoid any meal just before bedtime

Consuming just before bedtime, especially heavy meal, is prone to cause reflux problems. This is because the stomach has to produce great amounts of acid in order to digest the food.

The excessive acid tends to back up into the esophagus when you lie down. Generally, a good practice is to eat your last meal before 8 pm daily.

4. Avoid fast foods

Fast food is high in fat and will cause your stomach to produce more acid. Fast foods can also lead to weight gain, which will add to the problem of acid reflux.

5. Limit or avoid alcohol

Alcohol will add to the secretion of acid in the stomach. It may also curb the contraction of the esophageal sphincter. It is the failure of the sphincter muscle to contract tightly that leads to acid reflux.

6. Avoid frying foods whenever possible

Baked or broiled will serve two purposes; it will help control acid reflux symptoms and help to maintain a lower weight.

Do not drink alcohol in excess, especially fruit wines. Having a small glass of wine with dinner will probably be OK, but keep it to a minimum of one to two times a week.

7. Avoid foods that stimulate acid production

An acid reflux person should avoid foods that increase the secretion of acid in the stomach. These foods include coffee, spicy foods, tomatoes, citrus fruits, chocolate, and alcohol.

CHAPTER 7: UNHEALTHY FOOD COMBINATIONS THAT YOU SHOULD AVOID IF YOU HAVE GERD (ACID REFLUX)

Many people would want to know how to naturally cure their GERD, acid reflux, or any digestive disorder they have. They may have been tired of taking the same medicines prescribed by their doctor again and again, and have not achieved significant results.

This is why many are now looking for alternative means to relieve and if possible cure their condition. One of the ways is to practice proper food combining in order to bring your digestive system to heal and repair itself from one's past mistakes; one's unhealthy eating habits.

There are actually unhealthy food combinations that you should avoid, but 3 of these standout and these are usually the typical diet of most individuals:

1. Hamburger and Fries: You read that right. Knowing this truth might cost the regular fast food restaurants around your area a lot of profits, but your health is the issue here. We all know how juicy a hamburger is and how good it is to go with the fries. However, the basic problem here is that one is a protein and the other a starch, and these two should never be combined with any meal at any given time.

If you are suffering from GERD, acid reflux or any stomach ailment, think about the time when you were regularly taking your doctor's medication and still feeling the same lame results. Could it be that you just couldn't resist this type of food?

2. Spaghetti and Meatballs: Aaah yes. I won't be having any hamburger and fries, so I'll just go for my second best favorite, spaghetti, and meatballs! Surely that won't be any problem, right? Unfortunately, the same can be said for this delectable food combination.

Spaghetti is mostly made up of starch (and sometimes the sauce itself can aggravate your GERD or acid reflux), and meatballs are a concentrated type of protein. It's hard to admit, but these two are not just compatible with each other, although I know, they admittedly taste good together.

3. Eggs and Toast: For those of you who like to have this as one of your meal combinations every breakfast time, think again. You're better off starting out the day with a choice of your favorite fruits (alone) than thinking that eggs and toast would give you that much-needed boost of energy you need to get going.

Again, one is a protein and the other a starch. All three food combinations are just that tasty and some are even mouth-watering. You may even be caught up in the habit of making any or all of these three a regular diet. But the fact remains, they are a recipe for digestive disaster.

Digestive problems such as GERD are the number 1 reason people visit their doctors today. The tragedy is most people spend their whole lifetime in treatment and traditional medication, only to feel the same, or a lot much worse.

Hey, I myself felt like a lab rat undergoing trial and error approaches by my doctors and gastroenterologists, while they kept on burning a hole in my wallet.

CHAPTER 8: TREATMENT OPTIONS AVAILABLE FOR ACID REFLUX

Acid reflux treatment may differ from person to person, depending on the severity of the disease and the individual's body condition. Unfortunately, there isn't one fit of acid reflux cure for all. Acid reflux disease treatments can be classified into 5 main sections:

1. Changing your lifestyle as an acid reflux cure

In most acid reflux diseases, adopting lifestyle changes as a natural cure for acid reflux may be sufficient to control the pain and discomfort of acid reflux. The first step in treating acid reflux disease is to refrain from food that causes acid reflux. Other lifestyle changes include avoiding excessive eating, alcohol, coffee and smoking.

An overweight person may shed the excess pounds as a part of the acid reflux treatment plan. Since acid reflux symptoms can be worsened at night due to the lying position, raising the upper body by about eight inches while sleeping can give you a better sleep at night. Alternatively, you may choose to use an acid reflux pillow.

2. Over-the-counter acid reflux medicine

If lifestyle changes are not sufficient, you may have to resort to over-the-counter acid reflux medicine. Over the counter medications that are meant to treat acid reflux symptoms are common choices for millions of people daily. Products like Tums, Pepto Bismol, and Rolaids are convenient, cheap and don't require a doctor's prescription.

They function well in calming heartburn and other symptoms of acid reflux or indigestion. The widely available over-the-counter acid reflux medicines also included are antacids and H2 blockers. Antacids work on the principle of reducing the amount of acid in the stomach, whereas H2 blocker blocked the secretion of acid in the stomach.

When the acidity in the stomach is lessened, the occurrence of acid reflux reduces too. But, there are some harmful side effects that one should take note. Some of these are constipation or diarrhea, stomach cramps, or an increased thirst.

3. Prescribed acid reflux medication

In other chronic cases, a prescription acid reflux medication might be necessary. If medication is required for acid reflux treatment, it is likely that the acid reflux medication will have to be taken regularly and continued indefinitely.

These medications include prescribed version of H2 blocker and proton pump inhibitors.

4. Natural cure for acid reflux

The best natural remedy for acid reflux is still lifestyle changes as mentioned above.

Other natural cures may use herbal remedies for acid reflux such as herbal tea, cinnamon, pineapples, grapefruit and chicory root tea. Some people make use of homeopathic cure such as acid reflux and vinegar.

Eat bread, rice, and potatoes. These foods are always on the "do not eat" list because of their high carbohydrate count, but these foods do wonders for soaking up acidic fluids in your stomach.

This method doesn't require you to overeat carbs, but by having even one piece of bread, a half cup of rice or half a potato during a full meal, you can dramatically decrease the amount of acid reflux you experience after eating. One should always proceed with caution when using another acid reflux medicine.

ACID REFLUX SURGERY

For those who do not wish to depend on medication indefinitely, or the medication is simply ineffective, the last option is acid reflux surgery. Acid reflux surgery involves a laparoscopic procedure to wrap and suture the upper part of the stomach around the esophagus.

There is a small video camera on the end of a thin tube. This camera is inserted through a small incision in the belly button. The abdomen is filled with carbon dioxide to inflate it so that the surgeon can see.

The camera allows the surgeon to see the instruments. This puts the right amount of pressure on the lower esophageal sphincter. Patients are often discharged the same day as the surgery.

This is an easy, straightforward procedure that can relieve the pain of acid reflux. Recovery is generallyquick and such surgery has a good track record of successful cases. Acid reflux surgery is considered only when other options are exhausted.

In many cases, it is necessary to avoid further complications of acid reflux. Once surgery has been performed, it is a good idea to stick to a healthy eating plan that cuts out those foods that cause acid reflux. It would be a shame to counteract the effectiveness of the acid reflux surgery.

Basically, searching for the right cure for your acid reflux is an about knowing your symptoms and how they come together in your body and affect your system. When searching for the right acid reflux treatment, you should always think of the long term effect.

Never go for the short term relief and overlook about the long term implication.

CHAPTER 9: NATURAL REMEDIES FOR ACID REFLUX

Because prescription medications can sometimes have unwanted side effects, many people look for natural cures for acid reflux. In addition, most prescription medications were not designed to be taken for long periods of time, possibly while a person makes dietary and lifestyle changes which can be natural remedies for acid reflux.

Herbal remedies for acid reflux are based on what herbalists know of traditional medicine and traditional medicinal plants. Some of these are common food, herbs, which pose no danger for long-term use, but their effectiveness as natural cures for acid reflux has not been proven.

If you have been diagnosed with acid reflux, it is important to see your doctor regularly, even if you feel that your symptoms are under control. And you should let your doctor know about any botanical or herbal remedies for acid reflux that you may be using.

It is important to see your doctor regularly because stomach acid can damage the esophagus and lead to more serious conditions including cancer of the esophagus. If you are relying on natural cures for acid reflux and you become hoarse in the morning, develop a cough, or feel a need to clear your throat frequently, these may be symptoms of silent acid reflux.

Silent acid reflux is the term used to describe acid reflux that affects the voice box and the vocal cords but does not cause heartburn symptoms. So even if natural remedies for acid reflux keep your heartburn under control, you should still see your doctor regularly and report new or different symptoms.

Herbal remedies for acid reflux include chamomile, meadowsweet, slippery elm, cancer bush, fennel, catnip, angelica root, gentian root, ginger root and other botanicals, including aloe.

Slippery elm was used historically by native peoples to treat stomach upset, diarrhea, constipation, heartburn and other digestive complaints. Fennel and ginger root were also common "folk remedies" for the relief of indigestion. Modern herbalists have found that a combination of several of the herbs that had been used for indigestion could be effective natural remedies for acid reflux.

Some may call them natural "cures" for acid reflux, but the long-term relief of acid reflux is best accomplished by changes in lifestyle and eating habits.

For example, smoking relaxes the sphincter muscles that normally prevent stomach acid from reaching the esophagus. It also dries out saliva in the mouth and throat, which normally would neutralize some of the stomach acids and begin the digestive process.

If you use herbal remedies for acid reflux and you do not stop using tobacco products, then you may still have acid reflux and you are still at risk of developing esophageal cancer. The major risk factors for developing esophageal cancer include acid reflux, smoking, and alcoholism. This brings up another lifestyle change that is recommended for long-term control and relief of acid reflux.

Reducing or eliminating alcohol consumption can reduce acid reflux. In particular, alcohol consumption in the evening is believed to lead to more symptoms of nighttime acid reflux, as well as other health problems. While some argue that a glass of red wine has many health benefits, this is a 4-ounce glass, before a meal, and for those who suffer from acid reflux, even this may be a problem.

Alcohol increases stomach acid. Prescription and natural remedies for acid reflux are geared towards reducing or preventing excess stomach acid. It just does not make sense to continue to drink alcohol when you have been diagnosed with acid reflux.

Changing your eating habits may be natural cures for acid reflux. If you normally eat a large meal late in the evening, less than three hours before bedtime, then you are more likely to suffer from nighttime heartburn or other acid reflux symptoms like coughing.

This is because acid is traveling up out of the stomach and into the throat. Raising the head of the bed is also considered one of the natural remedies for acid reflux symptoms that occur at night. Gravity helps keep the acid in the stomach, but eating your last meal earlier and making it a smaller meal may prevent nighttime acid reflux.

Finally, weight loss should be mentioned as one of the natural cures for acid reflux. If you are currently at your ideal weight, then you may not need to read this section.

Overweight and obese people are much more likely to suffer from acid reflux, including nighttime acid reflux.

Trying herbal remedies for acid reflux control and making no effort to lose the extra pounds will undoubtedly be disappointing. Using prescription and/or natural remedies for acid reflux while you are trying to lose weight makes sense.

Avoiding fried and fatty foods are often recommended for people who suffer acid reflux.

If you avoid these and eat several small meals during the day, then you may naturally lose weight and naturally cure acid reflux.

Eating several small meals every couple of hours is often recommended by diet doctors, because it increases your metabolism and keeps blood sugar levels stable, so you don't feel sleepy after a meal, don't feel a need to lie down and stomach acid is less likely to travel back up into the esophagus.

CHAPTER 10: WAYS TO RELIEVE ACID REFLUX

The condition of acid reflux is also commonly known as heartburn. This is a condition that is characterized by the inflammation of the esophagus, caused by the backing up of food from the stomach into the esophagus. This food is partially or mostly digested and usually has a high acidic content, which causes pain and/or discomfort in many people.

Several treatments have been used successfully in the fight against heartburn (acid reflux). Some of these forms of treatment include one or more of the following:

1. Baking soda and water: Usually a teaspoon of baking soda mixed in a glass of water will help most people since it neutralizes excess acidity. This is one of the most natural ways to cure heartburn/acid reflux.

2. Alka-Seltzer: This is a tablet that dissolves in water that is taken orally as a liquid. This product has a similar effect as baking soda and water. It can be purchased at a pharmacy or grocery store without a prescription.

3. Pepto-Bismol: This is a liquid medication that is taken orally to help alleviate the effects of heartburn. This is available without a prescription.

4. Clear Soda (such as Sprite or 7-UP): The carbonation in clear sodas can help to relieve the acid buildup in a person's stomach and can also help a person to release gas.

5. Tums: These are tablets that come in a chewable form which contains calcium carbonate, an ingredient that helps relieve symptoms of upset stomach and heartburn. It is termed an antacid.

6. Prescription Medications: Those who need relief from chronic heartburn (acid reflux) can consult a doctor or otherqualified healthcare professional. They may prescribe more potent or different medications than those sold over-the-counter in stores. They will also provide instructions on how to take these.

7. Exercise: Those who engage in regular exercise will also find relief from heartburn in many cases. Usually, it is good to do a variety of aerobic and anaerobic movements.

Examples of anaerobic exercise involve fast-paced step exercises and dance movements, as well as jogging, stair climbing, and bicycling. Types of anaerobic exercise include weight and resistance training and stretching exercises.

More information can be found on specific exercise programs that can help people.

8. Diet Changes: If heartburn sufferers want relief, they may need to alter their diets.

9. Heat or Feet Pillows: Heartburn sufferers can also prevent or relieve acid reflux, particularly at night, if they raise their head or feet with pillows or another object (Such as a bed wedge).

Propping up the head usually works best since gravity can help keep food from creeping upward into the esophageal area.

10. Relaxation: If people take the time to rest and relax, they are better able to reduce the amount of stress that could lead to poor choices.

For example, it could reduce a person's desire to consume large amounts of alcohol, which can certainly aggravate the pain and discomfort associated with heartburn.

CHAPTER 11: TASTY RECIPES FOR PEOPLE WITH ACID REFLUX (GERD) FOR ORDINARY DAYS

Bad eating habit is the key ingredient in the recipe for acid reflux. An unhealthy eating lifestyle will most surely lead to acid reflux disease. Technically, acid reflux is known as Gastroesophageal reflux disease (GERD).

Acid reflux happens when excess gastric fluid or partially digested food backflow into the food pipe. Some common symptoms of acid reflux disease are chest pains and heartburn, where the sufferer experiences a burning sensation in the chest and throat.

Other symptoms include vomiting and sleeplessness. To ensure that you're eating habits do not contribute to the acid reflux recipe, there are a few simple rules to follow. First and foremost, do not consume too much in one meal. Eating too much causes the stomach to produce more gastric food.

It would be good if you could break food intake into five or six small meals a day instead of three huge meals. Do not eat two hours prior to bedtime.

If you really must, then have a small snack two to three hours before bedtime. This will give your stomach time to digest the food before you go to bed.

Next is to create an acid reflux diet. Like all food diet, there are the "good" foodstuff and the "bad" foodstuff.

Fresh fruits and vegetables will come under the "good food" list. However, it is advisable to avoid citrus fruits or juices as these may stimulate acid production in your stomach. Have some carbohydrates in your diet so that the gastric juices have something to work on. Observe moderation in each variety of food.

Avoid fatty meat, alcoholic drinks, drinks containing caffeine and carbonated soft drinks. All these "bad" foodstuffs are acid-stimulating. There are also other tips on reducing acid reflux, varying from sleeping position to posture and clothing. For example, it is believed that sleeping with the head slightly raised helps to keep the stomach juices from back-flowing into the esophagus.

The body of every human being reacts to different substances differently.

So make sure you consult your doctor and draw up an acid reflux disease prevention recipe that is ideal for your well-being.

1. ACID REFLUX BANANA TREATMENT

There are different ways to treat acid reflux symptoms, regardless of the cause. While some treatments involve the use of medications, other treatments take a more natural approach such as the acid reflux banana treatment.

Aside from being a really tasty and nutritious fruit high in vitamins and minerals, bananas contain virtually no fat, sodium, or cholesterol. For this reason, bananas are not only an integral part of a healthy diet, they can be used as a natural remedy to treat and prevent a number of health issues including, insomnia, depression, anemia, hypertension, and heartburn.

How exactly can a banana help with heartburn? Bananas have a natural antacid effect on the body. They primarily suppress acid secretion in the stomach by coating and protecting the stomach from acid, which helps against the formation of stomach ulcers and ulcer damage.

There are two ways in which the antacid property of a banana helps suppress acid:

Firstly, bananas contain a substance that encourages the activation of the cells that make up the lining of the stomach. As a result, a thicker mucus barrier is formed to provide the stomach with more protection against acid.

Secondly, bananas feature compounds called "protease inhibitors", which help to eliminate certain bacteria within the stomach that have been found to contribute to the development of stomach ulcers.

How can I add bananas to my diet? If you would like to help prevent heartburn by incorporating bananas, try eating a banana a half-hour before a meal, or directly after a meal. Some GERD (gastroesophageal reflux disease) sufferers also find eating a banana during a meal or half a banana before and after a meal beneficial. It's also a good idea to eat a banana when heartburn symptoms appear.

If the idea of eating a plain banana doesn't thrill you, there are more fun and tasty ways you can add bananas to your diet.

The following are some suggestions:

• Eat dried banana or mashed banana as a snack

• Cut up a fresh banana or use dried banana pieces and add it to cereal, yogurt, and salads

• Make a banana smoothie with live cultured yogurt

• Banana shakes (if you are allergic to milk and milk products, substitute with soy milk)

• Banana split - go easy on the ice cream

• Banana bread

• Banana muffins

- Banana cake

- Fruit bowl (excluding citrus fruits)

- Banana sandwich with cinnamon

Here are a few other facts to keep in mind when making banana recipes:

- Bananas with green tips are best used for cooking or should be left to ripen before eating.

- Bananas with yellow tips are best for eating

- Bananas that are browning or have dark brown or black specks are ideal for baking (Note: the riper the banana, the sweeter it will be because the starch has turned to sugar, making it better for baking)

- Bananas are the most popular fruit in America, are available all year round, and are low in cost, so it shouldn't be too difficult for you to make acid reflux banana remedies part of your regular diet. However, it is important that you eat bananas, according to your lifestyle requires. Keep in mind that Bananas are high in sugar.

Thus, if you are eating more than one banana per day, you do need to burn off the energy you are providing your body for maintaining a healthy body weight. Also, refrain from eating bananas close to bedtime because acid reflux can still occur when you are sleeping as the lower esophagus sphincter relaxes.

2. JUICER RECIPES

Juicing is a great way to make your diet healthier, and there are general rules you should follow to create your very own juicer recipes for energy. Juicing can be used to get the essential vitamins and minerals contained within fruits and vegetables without needing to actually fill up by eating them.

This book contains information about the beneficial effects of juicing and will guide you on how to create your very own juice.

If you want a healthy juice, choose a dark green vegetable for the base of your juice. You will want the juice to be between 50 to 75 percent spinach, chard, chard or something similar and make it at least half of what your juice is composed of.

This is what makes a "green smoothie" different from just a regular smoothie. These are the most effective ingredients for people who want to drink juice for health. Juices made exclusively from fruit often have more sugar and fewer nutrients than greens-based juices.

They can lend a bitter flavor to juice, however, so use them in conjunction with sweeter fruits or veggies, such as carrots, berries, and citrus. Fill the rest with your choice of fruits in order to achieve great taste. A popular berry blend is cranberries, blueberries, strawberries, and blueberries.

When you are juicing apples, use the ripest and sweetest apples that you can. If you decide to use bruised apples, make sure to cut the bruise off. Be creative and blend your own great-tasting juices.

After you're done juicing, immediately wash all the equipment that you used. Each of the fruits and vegetables contains different vitamins and nutrients. Wherever possible, make sure that you get the right nutrients while also making sure that you are able to enjoy a tasty drink.

Use cranberries as part of your juicing routine if you are having any bladder condition or urinary tract infection. Start adding them the moment you start to feel symptoms of a problem.

Pay attention to the cues your body's signals concerning the juices you consume. You may drink something that your system doesn't like. If you drink a new juice and feelqueasy or experience stomach churning, think about new fruits or vegetables you used in order to find the culprit. You can then use smaller amounts and condition your body to adjust to them.

Ginger is an all-natural remedy for soothing gastrointestinal issues. Ginger has many anti-inflammatory properties and can help with stomach ulcers and acid reflux disease or peptic ulcer disease.

If you are beginning to feel old and achy all the time, consider juicing as a great add-on to your life for a nice boost of energy! Juice offers several nutrients that may help assist your memory, aid memory or even slow down cell death due to free radicals.

As we said before, juicing is very good for you. When you juice, you get all the vitamins and minerals that are found in vegetables and fruits, but without the filling pulp.

By applying what you have learned in this article, you will be well on your way to juicing up your health. If you follow these principles, you will be well on your way to making your own delicious juice recipes for energy.

CHAPTER 12: GREAT HERBS FOR ACID REFLUX

Taking herbs for acid reflux may be a beneficial way to avoid heartburn so you don't ever have to worry about confusing heartburn symptoms with a heart attack. Herbs can help you stop heartburn before it starts which will help you limit the number of antacids or other medications you may take for heartburn relief.

There are various herbs used as health remedies, but only some are truly effective at preventing and relieving acid reflux. The following are 5 effective herbs for acid reflux.

1. Black Pepper: This is an aromatic herb that enhances taste, improves gastric circulation, and stimulates digestion. Black pepper can be added to recipes or can be an additional feature to prepared meal. For best results, use a small (approximately a tsp.) amount of fresh black pepper whole and grind it over food.

2. Indian long pepper: Indian long pepper is a powerful stimulant for digestion and is one of the most recommended for enhancing digestion, assimilation, and metabolism of foods ingested. In addition, Indian long peppers are fantastic herbs for acid reflux disease,

as studies have found it can provide considerable protection against the development of gastric ulcers.

Indian long pepper should be taken in small amounts (approximately a tsp.), and can be purchased dry and used in recipes, or added to meals for flavor. Simply crush the pepper to add it to food. Keep in mind that if you use too much, the flavor can become too intense, and you may find it too hot to eat.

3. Ginger: Ginger has been used for thousands of years to aid in digestion and treat stomach distress such as nausea, vomiting, and diarrhea. Ginger is one of the most highly effective herbs for acid reflux, and it is likely the purest. The effectiveness of ginger is due to its anti-inflammatory, antimicrobial and analgesic properties. Fresh ginger root can be added to recipes or added as an extra garnish to a finished meal. Ginger can also be taken in powder form and in tea.

Ginger is considered to be one of the safest herbal remedies to take, and you can ingest moderate amounts of it daily (I.E. tsp. of powder ginger, or an inch of a ginger root). However, be advised that if taken excessively, it may lead to mild heartburn.

4. Liquorice: Liquorice is a powerful herb and anti-inflammatory that studies have found are showing much promise as inhibiting the development of ulcers, wounds on the mucous membrane, and gastritis.

Liquorice also acts like an antacid. Liquorice was also found to improve the secretory status of Brunner's gland, which is located throughout the duodenum system.

Brunner's gland works to protect against the development of duodenal ulcers. Liquorice is available in powder form and can be taken in tea. A cup of tea or 3 tsp. of powder liquorice daily is considered safe to take. High doses of liquorice can lead to symptoms such as a headache, water retention, and high blood pressure.

5. Indian gooseberry: Indian gooseberry is a fruit that has been used to treat peptic ulcers and ingestion that is non-ulcer related. Studies have found Indian gooseberry to have considerable antioxidant effects, and it significantly reduced gastric mucosal injury and acid secretion. Indian gooseberry is made up of cell-protective properties as well as anti-ulcer, and anti-secretory properties.

You can eat an Indian gooseberry raw with a little salt, or you can take it in powder form and in the form of tea. This herb is not associated with side effects, but should still be ingested in moderation, as it can act as a laxative if eaten in copious amounts.

When considering herbs for acid reflux, keep in mind that you shouldn't take herbs as a form of medicinal treatment without first consulting your doctor about your plans. This is because some herbs may interact with other herbs, with medications you may currently be taking, or other health conditions you may have.

CHAPTER 13: TASTY ACID REFLUX RECIPES FOR 1 OR 2 WEEKS MUST READ

Curing oneself of the condition called acid reflux can be accomplished by using natural, healthy methods for some weeks. After a great deal of research I discover that with the proper use of herbs, health store items, meditation, exercise, and diet, one can heal themselves of acid reflux.

The first thing that I learned is that acid reflux, sometimes called GERD (gastroesophageal reflux disease), is not a disease at all. Contrary to what the medical community would have us believe, it is simply a condition, brought on by poor eating habits. Besides eating the wrong foods, not chewing food properly is probably the root cause of this ailment.

The Acid reflux condition would not exist without a damaged esophagus and a weakened LES (lower esophageal sphincter). If the condition is to be eliminated, healing the esophagus must be the first order of business. During this reflux recovery period, eating anything which could irritate or damage the esophagus, must be avoided.

Things like poorly chewed chips, crackers, cereal, or any hard foods with sharp edges are culinary culprits -

they cause little lacerations to develop in the esophagus. Until the lacerations have had a chance to heal, spicy foods, such as acidic tomato products, hot peppers, raw garlic and raw onions should also be eliminated from the diet.

They just further irritate the condition. Smoking and drinking alcohol relax the LES, allowing stomach acid to splash up into the esophagus, thus impeding the healing process. The key to acid reflux recovery is to eat only mild, easy to digest food until the esophagus has healed.

Eat early, giving yourself at least three hours of sitting or walking time before lying down. Eat slowly and chew your food completely. And last, but not least, try to eat in a relaxed, pleasant environment.

I have listed a few of my favorite recipes that I enjoyed during my own recovery period. They can be madequickly and easily. Try doubling these recipes so that you can reheat them later in the week; less time in the kitchen.

Remember that cooking from scratch, instead of relying on convenience foods, is a better approach to good health, in general. It is also nice to know what you are really eating. For breakfast, I believe that fresh fruit is the best way to go. I especially like melon and papaya.

For lunch, I eat more fruit like apples, bananas and, perhaps, some almonds, or walnuts. It's better to eat many little healthy meals during the day. I try to buy only organic fruits, however, sometimes when I am rushed, I purchase "ready to go" containers of mixed fruit at the grocery store. Try to stay away from pineapple, as I find it hard to digest.

How about starters in the evening? Serving vegetables raw is the ultimate healthy way to present them. Try creating a beautiful platter of crudité (crew di tay) better known as elegant rabbit food. Serve it with a savory tofu dip. Use cauliflower, broccoli, English cucumbers, radishes, green & yellow zucchinis, Belgium endive, carrot sticks, whole small mushrooms, or whatever appeals to you. Cut the vegetables into bite size pieces for dipping.

The Belgium endive is a natural, edible scoop for dipping. Just cut off the ends and peel off the leaves. Make the tofu dip by putting one package of soft or silken tofu in a food processor or blender, adding garlic powder, cumin, paprika and chopped chives or parsley for flavor and color. Season with salt & pepper to taste.

Add a little fresh squeezed lemon juice if the mixture is too thick. Process until smooth and creamy. If you are in a rush, ready made dips and raw vegetable platters are available in the produce sections of most supermarkets, but make a concerted effort to eat only organic, if possible.

I hope that you enjoy the following dishes. Even though I have cured myself of acid reflux, I still cook these recipes on a regular basis. I prefer food slightly undercooked. Feel free to adjust the cooking times and seasonings to your own taste. Bon appetite!

SAUTÉED WHITE FISH ON A BED OF MASHED POTATOES

This recipe is for one serving. Increase the ingredients for additional servings as needed.

One 4oz filet of white fish (orange roughy, sole, turbot, flounder, etc)

One med. Potato

Steamed green vegetable such as broccoli, spinach, peas or asparagus

Parsley or chives for garnish

¼ tbsp unsalted butter, olive oil or Pam

We will start with the potatoes because they take the longest to cook and they tend to retain their heat the longest. The fish and vegetable take only minutes to cook.

Peel and cube potato. Place in cold water to cover. Bring to the boil, and then simmer until fork tender. Drain, leaving just enough cooking liquid for mashing or whipping. You may also use the vegetable broth (recipe below) instead. Add salt to taste. Hold in a warm place.

Season fish with salt and pepper to taste. Place non-stick sauté pan over med high heat. Add butter, oil or spray with Pam. When notquite smoking, add fish. Cook two minutes, turn and cook other side for two minutes, or until the filet is lightly brown and cooked through. If the file is very thin, one minute on each side may be enough. (You can broil or bake the fish if desired)

Serve fish on top of mashed potatoes, surrounded by the steamed vegetables. Garnish with chopped parsley or chives.

VEGETABLE BROTH

This broth is very alkaline and rich in minerals. It can be served as a simple soup or used as a stock (as above) for cooking. Cook and save the potatoes and beets, use as a vegetable side dish or to add to soup.

2 cups red-skinned potato peelings

3 cups celery stalk

2 cup celery tops

2 cups beet tops

1 small zucchini or yellow squash

2 cups carrots

One small onion

Sprig of parsley

2 ½ quarts distilled water

Chop all vegetables into very fine pieces. Place in water and bring to the boil. Simmer for 20 minutes. Strain & refrigerate for future use.

Note: By cooking pearled barley in the finished broth with the addition of chopped vegetables, one can prepare a healthy soup for a first course.

PASTA PRIMAVERA

Primavera means "spring" in Italian. This pasta dish offers a great opportunity to use all the wonderful fresh spring vegetables at your disposal. However, you can make this dish anytime of the year by using whatever fresh vegetables you can find at your food market.

I have chosen a mixture of vegetables that I happen to love, for this recipe. You can use these or replace them with your favorites. During the reflux healing period, try to stay away from tomatoes, raw onions and raw garlic. I

have included garlic in this recipe (*see note regarding roasted garlic). If you can tolerate a little garlic, then make sure to cook it well at a low temperature, without browning it.

If you want to be a bit daring, you can add the optional cup of heavy cream. You may substitute parsley for the basil and the penne regatta for fettuccine, or other pasta. The whole family can enjoy this

Classic pasta dish.

1 cup sliced mushrooms

1 cup sliced carrots

1 cup baby peas

1 cup sliced asparagus spears

1 cup snow peas or sugar snaps

2 cloves garlic, finely chopped or roasted

1 lbs. Penne Regatta

1 tsp. Salt

3 tbsp extra virgin, first cold pressed olive oil

½ cup shredded basil

½ cup Parmigiano-Reggiano cheese

½ cup heavy cream (optional)

Place a steamer basket in a pot with a small amount of water and bring to the boil. Place vegetables in a basket, cover, and steam until tender (about 4 minutes). Rinse under cold running water to stop the cooking and preserve the color, and drain. To a large pot of boiling water, add salt and the penne regatta. Cook uncovered according to the instructions on the box, preferably al dente. Meanwhile, in a large sauté pan, heat the olive oil. Add the garlic and cook on a low flame for a couple of minutes (do not brown). Add the steamed vegetables and optional heavy cream and raise the heat to medium. Cook just enough to heat.

Drain the pasta and add to the sauté pan and mix well.

Sprinkle with Parmigianino Reggiano, and shredded basil. Heat the dish thoroughly and serve. If the dish needs more salt, use extra cheese instead, at the table.

Serve this dish with a heart of romaine salad with lemon chive dressing (recipe below)

* Note: It takes more than two cloves of roasted garlic, for this recipe. On a sheet of aluminum foil, place two heads of garlic and cut the stem end off with a knife. Drizzle a little olive oil over them and wrap tightly. Bake in a 400-degree oven for one hour.

When cool enough to handle, squeeze out the roasted garlic, into a bowl, discarding the shells. Mash well with a fork.

Another use for roasted garlic is my version of pesto sauce. I use walnuts instead of pine nuts, which I find indigestible, with the roasted garlic and basil. Use whatever proportion you like and drizzle first pressed, extra virgin olive oil into the blender. If your sauce is too thin, adjust with more walnuts, basil, and garlic. If it is too thick, use more olive oil. This is all a matter of taste. Serve with your favorite pasta. I prefer linguini or fettuccini.

LEMON CHIVE SALAD DRESSING

This is a simple, yet classic vinaigrette for green salads. Use heart of Romaine, Boston or Bipp lettuce. Make this dressing and hour or so before serving, in order that the chive flavor is fully incorporated. Remember to toss well before serving. The advantage here is using lemon juice, instead of vinegar. I find that lemon juice becomes alkaline after being ingested.

1 lemon juice

Sea salt (pinch)

3 tbsp. extra fine sugar

6 tbsp. extra-virgin olive oil

6 tbsp. minced chives (you can't have too many)

FRESHLY GROUND BLACK PEPPER

Combine lemon juice, salt, and sugar in a mixing bowl. Whisk until the sugar and salt are dissolved. Continue whisking in the olive oil, chives and several grinds of pepper. Keep whisking until dressing is emulsified. (Note: You can make this dressing for two by reducing the lemon juice to two tbsp, and the other ingredients by 1/3.) Keep leftover dressing in a jar in the fridge for future use. It will keep for about a week.

SAVORY LENTILS WITH TEXMATI BROWN RICE

1 lb of organic lentils (2 ½ cups), rinsed

8 cups water or stock

1 onion, chopped

3 cloves of garlic, chopped

2 carrots, sliced

2 stalks celery, chopped

1 bay leaf

2 sprigs of thyme or ½ tsp dried

Organic Texmati brown rice (follow instructions on package)

In a large pot, bring water and lentils to a boil. Add other ingredients. Reduce to the simmer, partially covered. Cook until tender (about 20 to 30 minutes), stirring occasionally and adding more liquid as needed. Remove the bay leaf and thyme sprigs. Season with salt and freshly ground black pepper to taste. Serve over organic Texmati brown rice. Garnish with chopped parsley. Serve with a light green salad, dressed with the lemon-chive dressing above.

BAKED CHICKEN BREASTS ON MUSHROOM CAPS WITH STEAMED BROCCOLI AND NEW POTATOES

6 chicken breasts (either bone in or halves with skin on)

1 tsp dried thyme

Olive oil

6 large Portobello mushrooms (or enough smaller mushrooms to cover the bottom of the baking pan)

1 tbsp minced garlic

Salt & pepper to taste

2 cups dry white wine or dry vermouth

¼ cup fresh chopped parsley

Place rack in center of the oven and preheat to 400 degrees.

Into a lightly oiled baking pan, large enough to hold chicken breasts, arrange mushrooms gill side down. Sprinkle with minced garlic, salt & pepper. Pour wine over the mushrooms. Place chicken breasts, skin side up, over mushrooms and brush with olive oil.

Bake uncovered about 20 minutes until the breasts are golden brown. If the wine has evaporated during the cooking process, add a little more (for those of you who can't tolerate alcohol, keep in mind that it burns off during the cooking process, leaving only the flavor).

Baste the breasts with the pan juices and turn over. Cook until breasts are completed done and springy to the finger, about 15 minutes more.

With a slotted spoon, place the chicken and mushrooms on a platter, mushrooms on the bottom and breasts on top, skin side up. Skim off excess fat and spoon juices over the chicken. Sprinkle with parsley.

Serve with steamed broccoli and boiled new potatoes. (Substitute brown rice for potatoes, if desired)

Stir fried shrimp and vegetables

Served over millet, brown rice or quinoa

3 tbsp Canola oil

1lb. raw medium peeled shrimp

2 cups broccoli florets

2 cups sliced mushrooms

4 scallions, trimmed and chopped

2 tbsp Garlic, minced

2 tbsp fresh ginger, minced

1 cup cold vegetable broth (see recipe above), mixed with 2tbsps, corn starch

1 package of organic millet

Into a hot wok or sauté pan, pour oil until just smoking

Add vegetables and stir constantly to cook al dente

Add shrimp and continue to stir until just turning pink

Add broth and cover for a couple of minutes until shrimp is almost done

Uncover and add cornstarch mixture, stir until thickened and turn off heat

Serve over millet cooked according to package instructions

Season to taste with tamari light soy sauce

Note: This dish must be done very quickly, as you don't want to overcook the shrimp or the vegetables. I have chosen Millet because it is an extremely alkaline grain. It is neutral in taste and will absorb the flavors of this dish. You may substitute brown rice instead.

CHAPTER 14: CREATING YOUR PERSONAL ACID REFLUX RECIPE

Acid reflux is a reality for many, and there are many reasons why it might happen. Though stress can be a problem, often the foods and drinks that people choose are the biggest triggers.

Things like alcohol, soda, spicy foods, fatty foods, and come citrus can bring about a world of pain for some. Some who have GERD-like to put together an acid reflux recipe book to keep track of the foods that don't bother them. Having such a book will make it easier for anyone with this condition to eat the right foods more often.

Before you begin compiling recipes, you should think about how you are going to store them. Your print can them out or write them down, but you may not be able to keep track of them that way. That means you probably aren't going to use them because you can't find them.

A simple three-ring binder is always a great idea, or you can use a box with index cards. These will keep all of your acid reflux recipes in one place.

When it comes to recipes, you might want to consider laminating the pages. This is extra work and an extra expense, but regular paper gets ruined very easily when in the kitchen. Laminating will help keep your recipes safe from grease, and they can be wiped off easily if something were to spill.

Finding recipes might be a matter of trial and error, but then there are tons to be found online. A simple search can dig up hundreds. You have to decide what you think sounds good. You can print them out and put them in your binder, or you can write them out on your index cards.

You should start with things that you know you would like, and then slowly add new things you would like to try. GERD sufferers should make sure their recipes are well balanced with proteins and carbs and should be low fat most of the time. Keep that in mind as you browse online.

Don't forget that you can also find great recipes by asking your doctor for recommendations. You can also find recipes by tweaking some of your favorite recipes that give you problems. You can also write them from scratch if you pay attention to what you can eat, and what is known to give you problems.

Things you should avoid would be citrus fruits, milk products (if you suffer from lactose intolerance), spicy foods, many sweets, fatty meats (buy lean cuts), and many forms of white potato.

Though taking the hot spices out of foods might sound like it makes for a bland diet, there are plenty of great herbs and seasonings that won't aggravate acid reflux. It might take you a while to come up with your own collection, but if you add a few new ones a week, your acid reflux recipe book will grow ratherquickly.

Though some of the foods that should be avoided bother many, they may not bother you. That is what will make your recipe book unique. If you don't have problems with spicy foods, then, by all means, include them.

There are no hard and fast rules for all people who have GERD. Even more important than what you eat is how you eat.

Remember to eat smaller and more frequent meals, and keep servings small, so your meals are not sitting in your stomach. That might be one of the biggest things to avoid.

CHAPTER 15: PERMANENT ACID REFLUX CURE

For those unfortunate enough to suffer from regular bouts of heartburn the possibility that there might be a permanent acid reflux cure will seem like the answer to their prayers. But, if you have an open mind and are willing to take an alternative view to solving your problem, your prayers will be answered.

This may seem a fanciful claim as the medical profession tells us that there is no permanent cure for heartburn and that taking some form of drug-based medication is the only way that we can control our problem. It is true that regularly popping those pills has brought that much-needed relief.

So is it possible that there is an alternative way to stop the pain and distress once and for all? The answer is YES and what is more, the cure does not rely on taking any drugs at all. But why are we told that there is no cure for heartburn and acid reflux? Quite simply, if somebody developed a product that could cure our problem, the pharmaceutical industry would lose a fortune in revenue.

Prescribed and over-the-counter medication for heartburn is one of the top money earners in the pharmaceutical industry, so where is the incentive to develop a cure? Cynical, but unfortunately true.

So if the pharmaceutical industry isn't going to provide the cure, where is it going to come from? Well, first of all, we need to understand that the conventional way of treating for acid reflux is to treat the symptoms and mask them by taking a pill.

This is why relief is only temporary. But this ignores a very important fact that acid reflux can be caused by many factors and variables, which include lifestyle, diet, environmental factors, inherited genetic traits, poor digestion, and toxins in the system. Simply dealing with the symptoms of heartburn will never solve the problem.

Doesn't it make sense that if you are going to cure your condition permanently, you must identify, treat and eliminate every one of the factors which are creating the problem? Of course, it does.

Once you have identified those specific factors that are causing your problem you can then set about dealing with them and eliminating them. Eliminate them and the problem will disappear for good.

The most effective way to achieve this is to follow a holistic program of treatment that combines strategic changes to diet and lifestyle with the most appropriate vitamin and herbal supplements. Totally natural and not a drug in sight! Treat the causes and not just the symptoms and you will have found the acid reflux cure which will give you that permanent relief from your heartburn.

All you need is the right guidance. Most conventional treatments for acid reflux and heartburn are temporary because they treat the symptoms and not the root cause of the problem.

So, if you want to successfully and permanently rid yourself of your heartburn then you must identify and address all the factors that contribute to the problem i.e. you must treat it holistically.

Part 2

Sweet Pea Smoothie

Total servings: 2

The Ingredients to Use

- 1 banana
- 1 ¼ cup of pineapple juice
- ⅓ cup of frozen peas
- 1 cup frozen strawberries

How to Prepare The Meal

1. Following the directions on the pack, prepare your peas. The, drain and rinse them.
2. Next, transfer the peas to a blender, along with pineapple juice, strawberries, and banana. Set the blender to high and process until it is smooth.
3. Pour the mixture into two glasses.

Beef Burgundy

Total servings: 6

The Ingredients to Use

- ½ pound of quartered mushrooms
- ⅛ pound of minced salt pork
- 20 peeled and trimmed pearl onions
- 1 diced large onions
- 1 ½ cups of beef broth

- 3 tbsp of flour

- 1 ½ cups of red wine

- 2 pound of cut stewing beef

- 2 bay leaves

- 1 tsp of dried marjoram

- 1 tsp dried rosemary

- 1 tsp of dried thyme

- ½ tsp of salt and ¼ tsp of pepper

How to Prepare The Meal

1. Using a casserole over medium heat, cook your salt pork. Once it is crisp, remove. Drain with a paper towel.

2. Add onions to the pork and cook till they are brown. Turn off the heat and roll your pork in a plate containing a mixture of flour salt and pepper.

3. In the same pot, brown your stewing beef and throw in your wine, herbs, and beef broth. Put your pork and onions back in the pot and cook for 1 ½ hours.

4. Put your mushrooms and pearl onions in the pot and cook for 30 minutes.

Stuffed Turkey Rolls

Total servings: 4

The Ingredients to Use

- 1 tbsp of soft margarine
- 4 turkey breast cutlets (¼ pounds)
- ¼ chicken broth, low-sodium
- 4 slices of low-fat and low-sodium smoked ham (1 oz)
- ¼ cup of dry white wine
- 2 slices of Swiss cheese (1 oz)
- 1 tbsp of mayonnaise, low-fat
- 3 tbsp of dry bread crumbs
- ½ tsp of ginger, ground
- Cooking spray, the non-stick kind
- 1 tsp of dried thyme

How to Prepare The Meal

1. Put pepper, a slice of ham, and ½ slice of cheese on each turkey cutlets. Roll the cutlets and stick toothpicks on each to hold them in place.

2. Add thyme and ginger to the breadcrumbs and mix. Coat your turkey cutlets in mayonnaise and sprinkle the breadcrumb mixture on them.

3. Oil a large skillet with cooking spray and set it over medium-high heat. Add your turkey rolls and cook for 5 minutes.

4. Pour your white wine, chicken broth, and add margarine to your skillet. Reduce the heat to low and continue boiling.

5. Cook for another 5 minutes and, once the sauce becomes thick, your turkey rolls are ready.

Mediterranean White Bean Soup

Total servings: 6

The Ingredients to Use

- Parmesan cheese, grated

- 1 tbsp of olive oil

- Fresh parsley

- 1 chopped large onion

- 2 cups of baby spinach

- 2 diced cloves of garlic

- 3 15 oz canned white beans, rinsed and drained

- 1 pkg vegetable broth

How To Prepare

.

- Add the beans, broth and other ingredients in large kettle

- Boil for 30 minutes more or until vegetables are tender

- Place into a bowl and sprinkle with Parmesan cheese. Sprinkle with seasoning as needed.

- Serve in a soup bowl and garnish to your liking.

Black Bean and Cilantro Soup

Total servings: 6

The Ingredients to Use

- 8 oz of canned beans

- 1 pint of chicken stock

- ½ cup of fresh Cilantro

- 1 tbsp of salt to taste

- Sour cream (non-fat)

How to Prepare The Meal

1. Boil the chicken stock. Do not over boil.

2. Add the beans, salt and the half cup of fresh Cilantro to the boiling chicken stock

3. Lower the heat and then boil all together for 30 minutes more.

4. Pour the boil into a blender and boil with a hand blender into the desired consistency.

5. Season as needed

6. Serve in a soup bowl and garnish it with 1 tbsp of nonfat sour cream and then add a sprig of cilantro.

7. You have a chocolate-like dish with green leaves on it and your cream by the side.

Cantaloupe Gazpacho with Flavor

Total servings: 2

The Ingredients to Use

- 1b. (2 cups) cantaloupe.
- The skin of the cantaloupe should be removed, and it should be seeded and cut into 1-inches pieces
- 2 tbsp of brown sugar
- Alternatively, use 2 tbsp of sugar
- Port wine
- Finely grated nutmeg in the relevant quantity

How to Prepare The Meal

1. Mix the cantaloupe, port, and sugar.
2. Stir together adequately and place in a freezer to be left for about 4 hours.
3. Take out after this and blend in a blender.
4. Finish with a dusting of nutmeg
5. Serve it immediately in a shot glass or small cup.

Creamy Hummus

Total servings: 4

The Ingredients to Use

- 1 can (19 oz.) of canned chickpeas.
- The chickpeas should be drained and washed at least twice
- 1 cup of chicken stock
- 2 tbsp of olive oil
- ¼ tbsp sesame oil
- ½ tbsp of sat.

How to Prepare The Meal

1. In a food processor, place the chickpeas with chicken stock, olive oil, sesame oil, and salt.
2. Process together until very smooth
3. Add chicken stock as needed to the smooth result.
4. Serve cold either with toast points, oven-toasted corn chips, or small wedges of flatbread.

Watermelon and Ginger Granite

Total servings: 3

The Ingredients to Use

- Seedless watermelon, well blended
- Get 3 cups of the blended juice
- 1 cup of water
- ½ cup of honey
- 1 whole clove

- A pinch of grounded nutmeg

- 1 tsp of fresh ginger already grinded

- 1 tsp of salt

- ½ tsp of lemon zest

How to Prepare The Meal

1. Mix the water, honey, clove, nutmeg, ginger, salt, and lemon zest and bring to a boil.

2. Allow cooling, then strain

3. Add the syrup to the watermelon juice

4. Place the juice in a bowl that can comfortably be placed in a freezer, then freeze for 4 hours.

5. Make sure to stir every 15 minutes with a sauce whisk.

Banana Sorbet

Total servings: 3

The Ingredients to Use

- 3 peeled bananas

- 1 tbsp of ginger. This should be peeled and grated fine.

- 1/8 tsp ground cardamom

- 1 tbsp of honey

- ¼ tsp of salt.

- 3 cups of ice

How to Prepare The Meal

1. In a blender, place the bananas, ginger, cardamom, honey and salt

2. Blend on high until very smooth.

3. Add ice and blend until creamy. Add more ice as needed to the creamy result.

4. Serve the result immediately or store it in a freezer

Carrot Salad

Total servings: 4

The Ingredients to Use

- 1 lb. carrots. This should be peeled, trimmed and grated

- ¼ 1b. Of mesclun greens

- 2 tbsp of raisins

- 2 tbsp of orange juice

- 1 tsp of dried oregano

- 2 tbsp of brown sugar

- 2 tsp of olive oil

- ¼ tsp of salt.

How to Prepare The Meal

1. Pour the raisins, orange juice, oregano, brown sugar, olive oil and salt in a bowl and mix. Leave the mixture to sit for about 5 minutes

2. Pour all over the carrots and mix thoroughly

3. Season all with additional salt as needed

4. Serve it over mesclun leaves.

Instant Polenta with Sesame Seeds

Total servings: 5

The Ingredients to Use

- ¾ cup of instant Polenta. Alternatively, you could use cornmeal instead

- 3 cups of whole milk

- 3 tbsp of brown sugar

- 1 tsp of orange extract

- ½ tsp of vanilla extract

- Get salt to taste.

- 1 tbsp of sesame seeds.

How to Prepare The Meal

1. Boil the milk. Don't over-boil

2. Add the Polenta or cornmeal and whisk forcefully to prevent any lumps in the mix.

3. Cook all again until cream

4. Add sugar, salt, and vanilla, and orange extract just before serving

5. Serve in a bowl, then sprinkle with sesame seeds.

Muesli - Style Oatmeal

Total servings: 3

The Ingredients to Use

- 1 cup of instant oatmeal
- A cup of milk
- 2 tbsp of raisins well boiled and drained before it is used
- ½ banana, well diced
- ½ golden apple. Well peeled and diced
- A pinch of salt
- 2 tsp of sugar, or alternatively 2 tsp of honey.

How to Prepare The Meal

1. On the evening before the day of preparation (or at least 2 hours before preparations), mix the oatmeal, milk, raisins, salt and sugar/honey together in a bowl.

2. Cover the mixture and put in the freezer

3. Add fruit before serving

4. If the mix is too thick (it should not be) add milk until it is free-flowing

Gala Apples Honey Dew Smoothie

Total servings: 6

The Ingredients to Use

- 2 cups of honeydew melon. Peeled, seeded and cut into chunks

- 4 tbsp of fresh aloe vera with the skin peeled off.

- 1 gala apple. The skin should be peeled, cored, and cut into half.

- 1/6 tsp of like zest. Use a grater to grate the zest

- One and a half cups of ice

- ¼ tsp of salt

How to Prepare The Meal

1. In a blender add the melon, ice, aloe vera, apple, salt and zest

2. Start blending on pulse, then switch to high after some time.

3. Stop and stir the mixture as needed to get a smooth consistency

4. Serve

Heartburn-Friendly Macaroni Salad

Total servings: 4

The Ingredients to Use

- 3 eggs, boiled hard.

- 2 cups of macaroni noodles of dry whole wheat

- 2 tsp of parsley cakes or alternatively, use 2 tbsp of parsley, fresh and finely chopped

- ¼ tsp of salt

- Ground pepper to taste. It should be freshly ground.

- 3 tbsp of mayonnaise. You can use either whole mayonnaise, low-fat or light.

- ⅓ cup of plain Greek yogurt (should be non-fat). Alternatively, you could use sour cream, but it must be non-fat.

- ¼ cup of finely chopped celery (optional)

- ¼ cup of finely chopped sweet or dill pickles.

How to Prepare The Meal

1. If you have not boiled your eggs already, then boil them. Following this, boil your noodles following the instructions on the noodles pack or simply boil for about 8 minutes.

2. Drain the noodles and simply leave to cool after you have rinsed thoroughly with cold water.

3.   Place the noodles in a bowl. Add parsley, salt, pepper and any other optional additions that are well-tolerated.

4.   Get a small bowl, pour your mayonnaise into it, blend your mayonnaise well, together with Greek yogurt then stir all into the noodle mixture left to cool and put in a serving bowl.

5.   Get your boiled eggs and peel the shell off the 3. Remove half of the yolks from the eggs, and chip the remaining eggs into the macaroni, then stir into the mixture.

6.   Cover it and let sit in the refrigerator overnight (if you have time).

Crispy Oven-Fried Buttermilk Chicken Strips

Total servings: 5

The Ingredients to Use

●   1 pound of chicken tenders

●   1 cup of buttermilk, low in fat

●   1 tbsp of canola oil to be used to grease the bottom of the baking sheet

●   ¾ cup of flour. Must be unbleached

●   ½ tsp of black pepper. Should be freshly cracked. (This is optional depending on if you can tolerate it)

●   ½ tsp of salt

- 1 cup of panko bread crumbs

- Canola cooking spray

How to Prepare The Meal

1. Thoroughly wash your chicken tenders and then dry them with paper towels. Get the pieces of chicken and mix them with the buttermilk. Place your mixture in a medium-sized coverable bowl and place in the refrigerator for 30 minutes or if it is prepared in the evening then leave in the refrigerator overnight.

2. Preheat your oven to about 400-degrees. After this, spread your canola oil thoroughly over a 9 × 13 inches baking dish.

3. If the above is ready then, get a shallow bowl and then place the flour, pepper, salt and cayenne pepper and whisk it altogether to blend the ingredients. Also, place the panko crumbs in a shallow bowl and then line up the bowls and pan in the following order: flour mixture, followed by chicken, add panko crumbs, then the prepared baking dish.

4. Next, take a piece of chicken, place it first in the flour mixture, then dip the chicken back into the buttermilk (this later exercise should be done briefly). Place your chicken in panko crumbs next, then lastly, place it in the prepared baking dish.

Repeat this exact process with the rest of the chicken pieces.

5. After the above, coat the top of the chicken strips generously with canola cooking spray.

6. Bake this in the center of your oven for about 25 minutes or more, depending on the intensity of the oven heat. Just ensure that the is nicely browned outside and well-cooked on the inside.

7. Remove from the oven and serve it with whatever sauce you desire or simply serve with condiments that are well-tolerated.

Spinach Artichoke Heart Dip

Total servings: 3

The Ingredients to Use

- 1 tbsp of olive oil, extra virgin

- 2 cups of milk. The milk should be low on fat (you can simply just use whole milk or fat-free milk).

- 4 tbsp of white flour (the white flour should be unbleached). Alternatively, you could use Wondra quick-mixing flour

- 1/8 tsp of nutmeg. This should be grounded nutmeg and it is optional.

- 1/8 tsp of pepper. This should be used only if tolerable, however, the pepper should be white.

- ⅓ cups of Parmesan cheese. The cheese should be shredded

- 10-ounce of packaged spinach. This should be frozen and chopped. It should also be thawed and squeezed to extract the excess water contained in it.

- 2 cups of artichoke hearts, well chopped. It should also be water-packed or alternatively, it should be thawed from frozen. Drain and chop it. You could alternatively use artichokes that are marinated. This should also be well-drained.

- 1 cup of skim mozzarella cheese. Use the shredded part.

How to Prepare The Meal

1. Turn on your oven and preheat it to about 350-degrees. Coat an 8×8-inch baking dish with canola cooking spray.

2. Next, make your Alfredo sauce if you have not done so. To make this, whisk together your olive oil, ⅓ cup of milk, 4 tbsp of flour, nutmeg, and pepper. In a nonstick saucepan, slowly stir your mixture in the remaining milk. Bring the mixture to a gentle boil over medium-high heat, then reduce the heat after some time to medium-low. Continue after this to boil gently, stir constantly until the sauce thickens. This should be done for about 2 minutes

or more. Stir in ⅓ cup of Parmesan cheese, which should be shredded.

3. After your Alfredo sauce is ready, add your garlic, green onions, spinach artichoke hearts, the prepared Alfredo sauce, and mozzarella cheese and bring all to a mix in a large mixing bowl and stir continuously with a spoon until it is a blend.

4. Spread the mixture above into an 8×8-inch baking dish and bake until it is bubbly. The baking should be done for about 30 minutes.

5. Serve warm with pieces of whole wheat (this should be bite-size). Alternatively, you could serve with sourdough bread or whole-grain crackers. Or better still serve with tortilla chips, depending on your preference

Chocolate-Free Blonde Brownies

Total servings: 3

The Ingredients to Use

- ½ cup of flour; whole wheat flour

- ½ cup of white flour. This should be unbleached

- ½ tsp of baking powder

- 1/8 tsp of baking soda

- ½ tsp of salt

- ⅓ fat margarine. This should be accompanied with 8 grams of fat per tbsp and there should be no trans fat

- ¾ cup of packed brown sugar. The brown sugar should be dark brown sugar.

- 1 large egg

- 1 tbsp of vanilla extract

- Mix-ins. This should be optional because it is not included in nutritional analysis

- Include ½ cup of cranberries, dried. Alternatively or in addition to the former, add ½ cup of walnuts or pecans and/or ½ cup of any other ingredients you add to your favorite chocolate brownie recipe. This recipe should, however, be something you tolerate well.

How to Prepare The Meal

1. Turn on your oven and preheat to about 350-degrees. Get a non-stick round or square pan or 9-inch. This should be treated with a canola cooking spray.

2. In a large bowl add flour, baking powder, baking soda, and salt into a large bowl and whisk together well and set this aside.

3. Place your non-stick saucepan over medium heat and melt your margarine in it. Stir it in brown sugar

and continue to cook for about one minute. Get the mixture from the heat and place aside to let it cool for a few minutes

4.   Get a large mixing bowl and add your brown sugar mixture to it. Add your egg and vanilla and beat on medium-low speed until all is well blended. Still, on a low speed add your flour mixture a little at a time and beat. Stir in the optional "mix-in" ingredients you have set aside. After this, spread it into a greased pan.

5.   Bake for about 20 to 25 minutes or alternatively until the brownies are done to your preference. If you like the brownies on the chewy side, don't overbake. Let it cool for about 10 minutes and cut it into 16squares.

6.   It is ready to be served.

Peanuts Butter and Raisins Banana Muffins

Total servings: 2

The Ingredients to Use

- 2 very large bananas
- 1 cup of steel-cut oats
- 1 tbsp of honey
- ½ cup of raisins

- ½ cup of smooth peanut butter. Smooth peanut butter is preferable because it is less likely to cause reactions

- ½ tbsp of baking powder

- Olive oil

How to Prepare The Meal

1. Turn on your oven and preheat it to 180°C, or to 160°C if your oven tends to burn food on higher temperatures.

2. In a large blender, mix the bananas, oats, honey, peanut butter, and baking powder. You can add some water to your mix if it's struggles in the blender. Pour the mix into a bowl after.

3. Add raisins and spread evenly throughout the mix.

4. Coat your muffin tray lightly with olive oil and then pour the mix into the muffin tray

5. Slide the tray into your oven and leave for about 2 minutes or leave until the mix is a golden brown color.

6. Remove and leave for some time to cool.

7. It is ready to serve.

Moroccan Kumara Breakfast Hash

Total servings: 2

The Ingredients to Use

- 1 large kumara

- 1 medium potato (a Desiree potato will be preferable). You could also use other potatoes of your choice.

- 1 bunch of broccolini

- 1 large green/red capsicum

- 2 tsp of Moroccan

- 2 large eggs

- Seasonings and Olive Oil

How to Prepare The Meal

1. Cube the kumara, Desiree potato, broccolini, and capsicum.

2. Place your wok on a stovetop with high heat. Set your frying pan on another burner with medium heat.

3. Add olive oil and drizzle some into your wok and on your frying pan. Crack your eggs into the frying pan and leave it to fry to your liking.

4. In your wok, drop your cubed vegetables and begin to stir with a wooden spoon

5. Add some Moroccan powder and mix it into the vegetable mix and begin to stir.

6. Place the lid on, and leave for about 20 seconds, then repeat the above process.

7. If the vegetables seem to be cooked and flavorful, then remove from the wok and put it into a plate. If it isn't cooked and flavorful enough, mix in some Moroccan powder again, stir and place the lid on then leave it for another 20 seconds.

8. Take out the vegetable mix place the fried eggs on top.

9. The recipe is ready to be served.

Garlic Parmesan Flaxseed Crackers

Total servings: 4

The Ingredients to Use

- 1 cup of flaxseed meal

- ⅓ cup of parmesan cheese. This should be grated

- $1^1/^2$ tsp of garlic powder

- ½ tsp of salt

- ½ cup of water

How to Prepare The Meal

1. Turn on your oven and heat it up to about 400 F. Then, get a silver con mat or greased parchment paper and cover it on a sheet pan.

2. Get a large bowl and get all your ingredients into it and then get some butter on to the prepared sheet pan with a spoon.

3. Use parchment or waxed paper to cover the mixture. Even out the mixture to about 1/8 inch. To do this you must not necessarily use a rolling pin. A ruler or a wine bottle could be used as alternatives. The most important thing is to ensure that in flattening it out, you don't allow it to be too thin around the edges. The effect of being too thin around the edges is that it will overcook before the center firms up.

4. After the above, remove the paper and then move around the edges with your finger to tuck the rough edges in and even it up

5. Place in the oven and bake for about 15 to 18 minutes. Ensure that the center is no longer soft.

6. If the product begins to get a little too brown around the edges, remove from the oven. If you want to cut it then you could cut into 12 even pieces either of square or rectangular shapes. Make sure to do the cutting before it cools off completely. Otherwise, you could just leave it to cool off completely and then it will begin to break into randomly sized pieces.

7. It can be served now.

Focaccia-Style Flax Bread Recipe

Total servings: 5

The Ingredients to Use

- 2 cups of flaxseed meal

- 1 tbsp of baking powder

- 1 tsp of salt

- 1 - 2 tbsp of sugar

- 5 eggs. Well beaten

- ½ cup of water

- ½ cup of oil

How to Prepare The Meal

1. Turn on your oven and preheat to about 350 F. Line a pan with oiled parchment paper or a silicone mat. A 10×15 - inch pan with sides will be best

2. Add all the ingredients together and in a large bowl whisk your flaxseed meal, baking powder, salt, and sugar.

3. Mix the beaten eggs, water, and oil. Stir together vigorously and combine with the dry ingredients. Ensure that the liquid part of the egg is not separate from the yoke.

4. Let the batter sit for about 2 to 3 minutes. This is important to allow it thicken up. Do not leave it for too long so that it does not get past the point where it is easy to spread.

5. Pour the batter into your prepared pan. To prevent it from forming a mound in the middle of the pan,

spread the batter away from the middles. Ensure the amount of batter in the middle is thin. You'll get an even thickness if you spread away from the center in a rectangle 2 inches from the side of the pan.

6. Bake this until it springs back when you touch the top. Or for about 28 minutes and/or when it is visibly brown.

7. Let it cool and then use a spatula to cut it into whatever size you want it. You do not necessarily need a sharp knife.

Free Almond Biscotti Recipe

Total servings: 3

The Ingredients to Use

● ½ cup of butter. It should be unsalted and at room temperature

● 3 cups of almond meal

● 1 tbsp of baking powder

● ¼ tsp of salt

● 1 cup of sugar substitute. Get a natural brand.

● 2 eggs.

● 2 tsp of almond extract

● 1 tsp of vanilla extract

How to Prepare The Meal

1. Turn on your oven and preheat to about 350 F. Use parchment paper or a silicone mat and cover it on a 10×15 - inch baking sheet. Lightly grease it with oil.

2. Get a large bowl and mix your butter, almond meal, baking powder, salt, and sugar substitute together. Beat until they are all fully combined and ensure that they completely together

3. Get your eggs and the two extracts and beat them into the mixture. Ensure that it is well combined with the earlier mixture. The batter should, however, be fairly stiff.

4. Leave the batter for about 5 minutes or more. The almond extract is expected to absorb the remaining liquid. It could end up absorbing only some. Just ensure that the result forms a soft dough that can be kneaded.

5. Turn the dough into the prepared baking sheet and form the dough into a rectangle of about ½ - ¾ inch high, 5 inches wide and ¼ inches long.

6. Bake this for about 22 to 25 minutes or until the top is very lightly brown in color. Remove from the oven and turn down the heat of the oven to about 325 F. Cut the cookies into slices of about ¾ inches wide after leaving the cookies to cool. Lay the slices on their sides and put them back in the oven for

about 15minutes until the sides have a slightly brown color.

7. You can leave the biscotti as it is or cut them into halves. Make sure to cool completely before serving. If it is not going to be served immediately, then store it in an airtight container.

Cheesecake with Almond Flour Crust Recipe

Total servings: 3

The Ingredients to Use

- 1 almond flour pie crust

- 16 ounces of cream cheese. This should be at room-temperature low-fat.

- 2 tsp of vanilla extract

- 1 tsp of lemon juice

- ¼ cup of agave syrup

- Salt to taste

How to Prepare The Meal

1. Turn on your oven and bake the almond flour pie crust. Baking could either be in a deep-dish 9-inch pie pan or 9-inch springform pan. Pat the crust mixture halfway up the side of either pan.

2. Use a medium bowl with a hand mixer or alternatively, a standing mixer. Combine your credit cheese, vanilla, lemon juice, and agave syrup into

the mixer. Increase the speed of the mixer to medium-high and beat for 5 minutes until smooth, light and fluffy

3. Spread out your cream cheese mixture into your crust and smooth off. Leave for at least 2 to 3 hours or until it is thoroughly cold and set.

4. It is ready to serve now. But before serving, run a knife around the edge of your springform pan and remove the collar. If you used a pie pan, this last step is unnecessary. Cover the cheesecake with fruit topping and serve.

Tomato Sauce-Free Lasagna Recipe

Total servings: 3

The Ingredients to Use

For pasta and beef;

- 12 ounces of wife lasagna noodles

- A pinch of salt to taste

- 12 ounces of lean ground beef. This could be ground round or ground sirloin

- A non-stick cooking spray

- ½ cuprous-sodium beef broth

Low fat Alfredo Sauce:

- ½ cuprous fat cream cheese

- 1¼ cups of milk. The milk should be skimmed or alternatively, 1% milk, divided

- 1 tbsp of an all-purpose flour

- 2 tbsp of butter or margarine

- ½ cup of shredded good-quality Parmesan cheese

- Salt and freshly ground pepper to taste

For Assemblage:

- 1¼ cups grated skim mozzarella cheese.

How to Prepare The Meal

Make the pasta and beef:

1. Preheat your oven to 325 F. Place a large pot of salted water on a stove and when it is boiled, add the lasagna noodles. Allow to boil well and drain.

2. While the noodles are boiling, spray a non-stick frying pan with oil and brown the beef

3. Ensure that your beef is well browned and add the beef broth and toss together until well-mixed.

Make the low-fat Alfredo Sauce:

1. In a large mixing bowl, pour in the cream cheese, ¼ cup of milk and flour. Mix together and add the remaining skimmed milk.

2. In a non-stick saucepan, melt the butter. While that is still heating, pour in the milk and cream cheese

mixture into it and stir. Your saucepan should be large and the heat should be medium. Continue to stir until the mixture is thickened or just simply leave on heat for about four minutes.

3. Add your Parmesan cheese and add your salt and pepper to taste and the stir.

The assemblage of Lasagna Noodles:

1. In a baking pan of about 13×9 – inches, spread one cup of the low-fat Alfredo Sauce on it. Lay 3 stripes of the lasagna noodles and spread half of the beef mixture on it

2. Lay another 3 stripes of lasagna noodles on the mixture and then spread the remaining beef mixture and then lay another 3 strips of lasagna noodles on it.

3. Spread the remaining cup of Alfredo Sauce on the mixture and sprinkle your mozzarella cheese and leave to bake in the oven for about 35 minutes. Just ensure that the result is bubbly and golden.

Almond Flour Gluten-Free Muffins

Total servings: 6

The Ingredients to Use

- 2 cups of almond flour

- 2 tsp of baking powder

- ¼ tsp of salt

- ½ cup of apple sauce

- 5 large eggs. Should be room-temperature beaten

- ⅓ cups of water

- 5 tbsp of agave syrup

How to Prepare The Meal

1. Turn on your oven and heat it to about 375 F.

2. Coat a 12-cup muffin pan with cooking spray. In a large bowl pour in your almond flour, baking powder, and salt and beat all together until it's well mixed.

3. In a separate medium bowl, mix your apple sauce together with eggs, water, and agave syrup. Mix all thoroughly but not too much. If mixed too much it could result in what is known as 'tunneling.'

4. Use any pan of your choice and scoop your muffin batter into it. Fill each about ⅔. Bake it in the oven for about 15 minutes. To determine if it is ready, dip a toothpick into it and drag out. It is ready if the toothpick comes out clean.

5. Remove from the oven and wait for about 5 minutes or more. Then invert muffins to a wire rack. You can eat your muffins warm or at room temperature.

Low- Carb Lemon Ricotta Pie

Total servings: 4

The Ingredients to Use

- 1 pound of whole milk ricotta cheese. A 15-ounce container will be better

- 3 eggs

- One medium-sized lemon. Juice and grated zest

- Sugar substitute which should equal ⅔ cup of sugar. Zero carbs are preferable as liquid sucralose

- ½ tsp of vanilla extract

- Salt

How to Prepare The Meal

1. Turn on your oven and preheat to about 350 F.

2. Break your egg and separate the yolk and then beat the white part into a soft peak for.

3. Add the egg yolks and the rest of the ingredients. Taste the mixture to ensure it is lemony enough. This is because some lemons are "dryer" than others and as such have less juice. An average lemon should be about 3 tbsp of juice for a medium-sized lemon. Depending on your preference, you could add half a tsp of lemon extract or more lemon juice to taste

4. Fold egg whites into the mixture. In a pan, spread your butter, then spread the mixture.

5. Bake it until it is barely set. Or simply bake for about 25 minutes

6. Allow it to cool completely before serving. Perhaps about 90 minutes after removing from the oven. You can serve plain or serve with toppings such as strawberry toppings or berry syrup. You can also use sugar-free lemon toppings, this comes as a very good topping.

Gluten-Free Fresh Berry Pie

Total servings: 5

The Ingredients to Use

For the Almond Pie Crust:

- 3 tbsp of butter

- 1½ cups of almond meal. Alternatively, use almond flour

- 2 tbsp of agave. Alternatively, use honey

For the berry pie filling:

- ¾ cup of water

- 4 cups of fresh blackberries

- Salt
- ¾ cup of honey or simply use other liquid sweeter

- 4 tsp of cornstarch

- Optionally you can add 1 tbsp of butter. This is highly recommended.

- Optionally, you can also add whipped cream for serving.

How to Prepare The Meal

Make the almond piecrust:

1. Turn on your oven and pre-heat at 350°F.

2. In a microwave-safe pie pan, melt the butter, then pour in your almond meal and agave into the melting butter and mix gently. Use your finger to pat it.

3. Place in the oven and leave it to bake for about 10 minutes until the crust is brown in color. Take note that after 8 minutes of the mixture staying in the oven, you have to check it every other minute to ensure that it does not over-brown.

Make the berry pie filling:

1. In a large bowl, add water, berries, salt, and honey.

2. Bring to a boil for about 3 minutes. Boil until the berries soften and the liquid is a very-like color

3. Get your cornstarch and whisk it into the mixture. Allow boiling until the cornstarch softens and the liquid darkens and clarifies.

4. Add your butter next (if you are making use of butter) and then add your remaining berries into it and stir it.

5. Pour the mixture into the baked almond pie, which should be cooled.

Vegan Grain Bowls with Mediterranean Chimichurri

Total servings: 3

The Ingredients to Use

- 2 medium-sized zucchini
- ½ tsp of pepper
- 1 tbsp of olive oil
- 1⅓ cup of whole wheat orzo
- 1 can of low sodium chickpeas
- 12-ounces jar of roasted red pepper
- ¼ cup of pine nuts
- 1 shallot. Should be finely chopped
- 4 garlic cloves. Should be minced
- 1 tsp of salt
- ½ cup of fresh basil
- 1 tsp of dried oregano
- ¾ cup of extra virgin olive oil

- ½ cup of fresh parsley

- ¼ cup of red wine vinegar

- ¼ cup of water

How to Prepare The Meal

1. Chop the zucchini into bite-sized pieces. Toss into pepper and olive oil and roast at about 470 F for about 25 minutes.

2. Add Chimichurri ingredients into either a food processor or a blender and then blend until it is finely chopped.

3. In a pot of boiling water, add your orzo and leave it for about 8 to 9 minutes and then sieve out in a colander. Pour it back into the pot and then mix it with about 2 spoons of the Chimichurri mixture to prevent it from sticking.

4. Drain your chickpeas and rinse thoroughly.

5. In a large bowl mix your orzo, zucchini, pepper, chickpeas and artichoke hearts together and sprinkle with Chimichurri sauce and add your pine nuts.

Low-Carb Banana Bread Recipe

Total servings: 4

The Ingredients to Use

- 3 medium bananas. Should be very ripe

- 3 large eggs

- 2 tbsp of oil

- 2 cups of almond meal

- 1 tbsp of baking powder

- ½ tsp of salt.

How to Prepare The Meal

1. Turn on your oven and preheat to about 370 F

2. Get a loaf pan of about 9×6 inches and lightly coat it with oil spray and set it aside.

3. Gently mash your bananas and fill them out into two measuring cups. It is not important that the bananas fill the two measuring cups. In fact, it should not. Only ensure that all your wet ingredients the measuring cups.

4. Next thing you break your egg into the measuring cups and add your oil and then turn gently with a fork until the whole content of the measuring cup is a blended mix then add water into the measuring cup to fill it to the brim.

5. Get a separate bowl and then mix your almond meal, salt and baking powder together and then pour the liquid content into the dry content and mix together for about 3 minutes. Ensure that you do not overmix the ingredients.

6. Next step is to pour out the mixture into the pre-prepared loaf pan and spread it until the top is opened out then put in the oven and leave it to bake for about 55 minutes or less or just simply until the toothpick theory is applicable

7. Bring it out from the oven and allow it to cool before placing it on a wire rack. Use your knife next to go round the edges and then turn it to the other side for it to cool entirely before you can cut into any pieces and then serve.

Greek Yogurt with Walnuts and Honey

Total servings: 6

The Ingredients to Use

- 4 cups of Greek yogurt. Should be free from fat and could be plain or vanilla

- ½ cup of California walnuts. Should be chopped and toasted

- 3 tbsp of honey. Alternatively, use agave nectar

- Fresh fruits. It should be well chopped. Alternatively, use granola. This should be low fat. (They both are optional but highly recommended)

How to Prepare The Meal

- Spoon your yogurt into the various cups

- Add walnuts and sprinkle 2 tbsp on each cup. Drizzle 2 tsps of honey on each cup

- Add the fruit or granola if desired.

Seeded Walnuts Lavosh Crackers

Total servings: 5

The Ingredients to Use

- 1½ cups of flour

- 2 tbsp of sugar

- 6 tbsp of everything that is a bagel. It should be seasoned and divided also.

- ½ tsp of sea salt or fine smoked sea salt

- ¼ tsp of baking soda

- ¼ cup of butter. Should be softened

- ½ cup in addition to 2 tbsp of buttermilk. Should be divided

- ¾ cup of finely chopped California walnuts. This should also be divided

How to Prepare The Meal

1. Turn on your oven and preheat to about 375°F. Stir together sugar, flour, salt, baking powder and 4 tsp of bagel seasoning in a large bowl. After mixing for some time, add your butter and half a cup of walnuts and mix this time around with a form.

Further, add half a cup of buttermilk and stir until it is well mixed.

2.   Bring the mixture to a flat surface (a lightly-floured board) and knead the mixture several until it is fluffy and forms a small ball. Divide the ball into 4 equal parts and then roll 2 parts as think as you can on a floured board. Place it on a parchment-lined baking sheet and brush it with buttermilk. Set apart. Sprinkle each with walnuts and bagel seasoning. Press lightly with your fingertips.

3.   Bake for about 18 minutes or alternatively until it is a light golden brown. Repeat this process with the remaining 2 parts left. Cool completely and break each into half, and the half into pieces.

4.   Serve.

Chorizo White Bean Soup

Total Servings: 6

The Ingredients to Use

- 2 chopped medium carrots
- 2 tbsp of olive oil
- 3 minced garlic cloves
- 1 pound of chorizo sausage (remove the casing)
- 1 tsp of kosher salt
- 1 tsp of paprika

- ½ cup of fresh, chopped parsley leaves

- ½ pound of chopped small red potatoes.

- 2 cans of cleaned and rinsed Great Northern beans

- 1 container of reduced-sodium chicken broth

How to Prepare The Meal

1. Set your Dutch oven to medium-high. Cook the chorizo while stirring until it is crumbled and brown for about 8 minutes. Use a paper towel to drain it properly and clean the Dutch oven.

2. With the Dutch oven set to the same medium-high heat, heat the oil. Sauté onions and the other ingredients until they are soft. Add the tomato paste and cook for one minute with continuous stirring.

3. Change the heat to high. Boil a mixture of chicken broth, beans, and chorizo. Bring back the heat to medium-low. Allow it to simmer for 20 minutes while you stir and skim off fat accumulating at the top, at intervals. Add the parsley, stir, and serve at once.

Whole-Wheat Pasta With Mushrooms

Total servings: 1-2

The Ingredients to Use

- 12 ounces whole-wheat pasta

- 1 sliced shallot

- A pinch of garlic salt

- 4 ounce of packaged pre-sliced mixed mushroom

- 16 ounce of packaged pre-sliced shiitake mushroom blend

- 16 ounce of packaged pre-sliced baby portobello mushrooms

- 2 tbsp of freshly chopped parsley

- ⅓ cup of freshly chopped parsley

- ⅓ cup grated Parmesan

- 1 ½ tbsp truffle oil

How To Prepare The Meal

1. Boil a large quantity of water in a pot. Add a little garlic salt and follow the directions to cook pasta.

2. ½ tbsp of olive oil should be heated in a large nonstick pan and used to sauté the shallot. Place in the mushrooms and cook them for 5-6 minutes at medium-high heat or until they turn brown. Once brown on one side, flip over for another 5-6 minutes until brown on the other side. Add ¼ tsp pepper and ½ tsp salt.

3. Drain out the pasta and mix it with the mushroom in a large bowl. Pour in the remaining 1 tbsp of olive oil, the truffle oil, and the salt and pepper. Stir the mixture.

4. Serve it hot with Parmesan and parsley as the toppings.

Raisin Pecan and Carrot Bread

Total servings: 1-2

The Ingredients to Use

- 1 tsp of baking soda
- 2 eggs
- ⅔ cup of whole wheat pastry flour
- ⅓ cup of chopped pecans
- 1 cup all-purpose flour
- Orange zest
- ⅓ cup of raisins
- 1 tsp of ground cinnamon
- 1 tsp of vanilla extract
- 2 tbsp of plain Greek yogurt
- 1 heaping cup of grated carrots
- 1 tsp of vanilla extract
- ¼ tsp of salt
- ¾ cup of granulated sugar

How to Prepare The Meal

1. Set your oven to 350°F to preheat it.

2. Grease a standard-sized loaf pan with cooking spray or butter and place parchment paper on the bottom.

3. Sift the flour, baking soda, salt and cinnamon into a medium bowl. Beat eggs, sugar, and oil until it is light and fluffy in a large bowl. Then add the grated carrots, Greek yogurt, orange zest, and vanilla, then stir. Mix all the dry ingredients and add the chopped pecans and raisins.

4. Turn the batter into the prepared loaf pan and allow it to bake for 45 minutes or when you can insert a toothpick into the bread center without sticking.

Vegan Coconut Rice Pudding

Total Servings: 6

Ingredients to Use

- 1 cup of brown or white rice
- 1-15oz canned full fat coconut milk
- 2 tbsp of vanilla extract
- ¼ cup of maple syrup
- 1 cup of raisins
- 2 tbsp of cinnamon
- 1 cup of unsweetened almond milk
- Pinch of salt
- The toppings

- Coconut Whipped cream
- Blueberries
- Cinnamon sprinkles

How to Prepare The Meal

1. Using a medium-sized saucepan, boil one can of full-fat coconut milk

2. Add the boiling coconut milk to a properly washed and drained rice.

3. Boil it for 5 minutes, cover and allow it to simmer for 20 minutes.

4. Stir and mix in the cinnamon, vanilla extract, 1 cup of almond milk and maple syrup. If you are using raisins, add them.

5. Cook again for 10 minutes. Add another ½ cup of almond milk, If you still want the rice to be creamier.

6. Stir at intervals to avoid rice sticking to the pan's bottom. You can also add more cinnamon if you think you want more

7. Turn off the heat and allow it to cool for 5 minutes. Add the toppings and eat from glass cups or bowls. If you do not want to eat immediately, store in a fridge until it gets cold. If you still want more creaminess, pour more almond milk on it.

8. For storage, preserve in a fridge in airtight containers for about 4 days and heat before you serve, if you wish.

Creamy Zucchini Quiche

Total servings: 6

Ingredients to Use

- 2 tbsp of butter
- Salt
- 3 cups of grated zucchini
- ½ cup of whipped cream
- 1 pie shell (9 inches), unbaked (9-10 inch)
- 8 large sliced mushrooms
- Salt and black pepper
- 2 tbsp of Dijon mustard
- 2 cups of Monterey Jack cheese
- 8 ounces of cream cheese
- 2 egg yolks

How to Prepare The Meal

1. Use mustard to coat the bottom of a pastry shell.
2. Set the oven to 450°F (230°C) and bake for 10 minutes.

3. Cool and set the oven heat at 350°F (180°C).

4. Sprinkle the salt on zucchini in a colander and drain for 5 minutes. Then sauté the mushrooms in butter.

5. Fill the bottom of the pastry shell with 1 cup of Jack cheese and place mushrooms on it.

6. Remove the extra moisture from the zucchini by squeezing it, after which you separate with your fingers.

7. Mix the cream, cream cheese, egg, and egg yolks. Add the pepper and salt.

8. Set the pastry dish upon a baking sheet and meticulously put in the egg-cream mixture. Then arrange the remaining Jack cheese at the top.

9. Set the oven to 350°F (180°C) F and bake for 45 minutes. The top will become golden and puffed and a toothpick inserted will not stick. Let it stand for five minutes before you cut.

Ginger Snap Beef Stew

Total Servings: 5

Ingredients to Use

- 1 tbsp of vegetable oil

- 1½ cup of water

- 1 bay leaf

- 1¼ pound of lean, trimmed beef stew meat (diced into 1-inch pieces)

- ¼ cup of white vinegar

- 1 large thinly sliced onions

- ¾ tsp of caraway seeds

- ½ tsp salt

- 1 tbsp of sugar

- ½ small red cabbage chopped into 4 wedges

- ⅛ tsp of ground black pepper

- ¼ cup of crushed gingersnap

How to Prepare The Meal

1. Pour oil in a heavy skillet and use it to brown meat. Replace the meat with onion and sauté until it is golden, in the remaining oil.

2. Put the meat back in the skillet. Mix the bay leaf, caraway seeds, pepper, water, and salt. Boil the mixture. Cover it and allow it to simmer with low heat for 1¼ hours.

3. Stir in sugar and vinegar. Arrange the cabbage on the meat, then cover and let it simmer for another 45 minutes.

4. Place the meat and cabbage on a platter so it stays warm.

5. Skim the fat of the drippings after straining. Pour into the drippings enough water to produce 1 cup of liquid. Mix the gingersnap crumbs and drippings in the skillet. Cook and stir while letting it boil and thicken.

6. Cover the vegetables and meat with sauce.

Baby Kale and Edamame Salad

Total servings: 4

Ingredients to Use

for the dressing:

- 1 tbsp of honey
- ¼ cup of soy sauce
- 2 tbsp of fresh lemon juice
- 1 tbsp of minced fresh ginger
- ¼ cup of toasted sesame oil
- 2 cloves of garlic
- 1 tbsp of hot sriracha or fix sauce

For the salad:

- 4 cups of torn kale leaves
- 3 chopped green onions
- 1 cup of shelled, cooked edamame
- 1 cup of chopped fresh cilantro

- 1 tbsp of sesame seeds

- 2 large carrots sliced into thin ½ moons

- 2 sliced bell peppers

- ⅔ cup of cashews (toasting is optional)

- 1 cup of shredded purple cabbage

How to Prepare The Meal

1. Mix and blend all the dressing ingredients until it is smooth then put it apart.

2. Follow the instructions to cook the edamame. Shell it after allowing to cool into you get 1 cup.

3. Drizzle the torn kale with some oil. Massage it for about 3 minutes until it is a little softened.

4. Mix all the salad ingredients. Add the dressing and toss. Serve at once.

Tip:

You can toast your cashews easily if you set your skillet on medium and cook till they are golden brown.

Butternut Squash Soup

Total Servings: 8

Ingredients to Use

- Olive oil

- 2 carrots

- 2 sticks of celery

- 16 fresh sage leaves

- 2 red onions

- 2 kg butternut squash, Mosque de Provence, onion squash

- 4 garlic cloves

- ½ - 1 fresh red chili

- Extra virgin olive oil

- 2 liters vegetable stock or organic chicken

- 2 sprigs of fresh rosemary

- For the Croutons

- Parmesan cheese

- 16 slices of ciabatta bread

- Extra virgin olive oil

How To Prepare The Meal

1. Peel the carrots, onions and garlic, then chop them. Chop the celery finely after trimming. Feared the chili, pick the rosemary and chop them.

2. Use a large saucepan to heat some lugs of olive oil over medium heat. Fry the sage leaves in it for 30 seconds. Remove the kitchen paper when it is crisp.

3. Cook the carrot, chili, Garlic, onion, celery, rosemary, black pepper, and a pinch of sea salt

gently for about 10 minutes. It will become soft and sweet.

4. Divide the squash into two and deseed and chop it up. Mix the squash and stock together in the pan and boil it at a simmer for 30 minutes.

5. To make the crouton, rub the ciabatta with a little olive oil. After patting it in, grate finely some of the Parmesan and press it into each side. Fry it in a dry, nonstick pan, let the sides turn golden.

6. As soon as the squash is tender, use a stick blender to turn the soup or use a blender to pulse it to a smooth purée. If you like it chunky, then you can leave it that way.

7. Add the salt and pepper to your taste. Share it between bowls and put 2 croutons on each.

8. Spread some crispy sage leaves. After that sprinkle some twirl of extra virgin olive oil. Serve.

Tips

This soup can be made in different ways when you have mastered it. All you should do is add dried pasta, pearl barley and even chopped smoked bacon. If you want you can add a tiny dried porcini.

Orecchiette with Brussels Sprouts and Hazelnuts

Total Servings: 6-8

Ingredients to Use

- ½ tsp of kosher salt

- 2 tsp of minced garlic

- ¾ pound of trimmed and halved Brussels sprouts

- ¼ cup of chopped toasted hazelnuts

- 1 ounce of finely diced pancetta

- 1 tsp of minced fresh thyme

- 1 tbsp plus 2 tsp of extra-virgin olive oil, divided

- ¼ tsp of freshly ground black pepper

- 3 tbsp of freshly grated Parmesan

- 8 ounces of dried orecchiette pasta

How to Prepare the meal

1. Heat the oven to 425°F. Use 1 tbsp of oil to toss the sprouts and cut on a baking sheet. Spray some pancetta, pepper, and salt. Roast the sprouts for 18-20 minutes until they become tender.

2. Cook the pasta by following the instructions. Drain the pasta and remain ¼ cup of the cooking water. Then place the pasta back in the pot.

3. Mix the garlic in the sprouts. Add the Parmesan, sprouts, thyme and some tbsp of reserved pasta water to the pasta. Pour in the 2 tsp of oil remaining. Put into 4 bowls and arrange the hazelnuts on top.

Peachy cobbler

Total Servings: 6-8

Ingredients to use

- 3 tbsp of lemon juice
- 1 tsp of cinnamon
- ¼ tsp salt
- ¾ cup all-purpose flour
- 4 ripe peaches or one bag of frozen sliced peaches
- ¾ cup of milk
- ½ cup of Redi measure light brown sugar
- 6 tbsp of unsalted melted butter
- ½ cup of Imperial sugar extra fine granulated
- 2 tsp of baking powder

Garnish

- ½ pint of raspberries
- 1 peach

How to Prepare the meal

1. Set the oven at 350°F
2. If you are using fresh peaches, slice them evenly and arrange on the bottom of a bake-proof pan of 9 x 9 inches.

3. Sprinkle with brown sugar and cinnamon when you pour it on lemon juice.

4. Sift flour and baking powder in one bowl. Mix in sugar and salt. Whisk in the milk until it is smooth.

5. Mix the cake batter to a thin consistency and spread over the peaches. Also, spread melted butter and put it in the oven. Let it bake until the center becomes golden brown and rebounds after being touched with a finger. This may take 35-40 minutes.

6. Remove from the oven and glitz it up with fresh raspberries and peaches, and confectioner's sugar.

Roasted Vegetable Lasagna

Total Serving: 10

Ingredients to Use

- Kosher salt and ground black pepper

- 1½ pounds of unpeeled eggplant sliced lengthwise ¼ inch thick

- 16 ounces of fresh whole-milk ricotta

- ¾ pound of unpeeled zucchini, sliced lengthwise ¼ inch thick

- 10 ounces of lasagna noodles

- 2 extra-large eggs, beaten lightly

- ⅔ cup of good olive oil

- 1 cup of freshly grated Parmesan cheese (divided)

- 1 tbsp of dried oregano

- 1 pound of very thinly sliced lightly salted fresh mozzarella

- ½ cup of chopped fresh basil leaves, lightly packed

- 8 ounces of creamy garlic and herb goat cheese stored at room temperature

- 1 tbsp or 3 cloves of minced garlic

- 4½ cups good bottled marinara sauce

How to Prepare The Meal

1. Set the oven at 375 degrees. Line 3 sheet pans with parchment paper and arrange zucchini and eggplant on them in single layers. Use a large quantity of olive oil to brush on both sides. Add the 1½ tbsp of pepper and 1 tbsp of salt, then sprinkle the oregano. Sprinkle the garlic on the vegetables after the first roast of 25 minutes. When that is done, roast again for 5 minutes until the vegetables become soft. After removing it from the oven turn the heat down to 350°F degrees.

2. Boil water in a very large bowl. Make sure the temperature is at 140°F degrees. Put the noodles inside the water one after each other and allow them to soak for 15 minutes. Stir at intervals to prevent sticking. Drain the noodles and twirl.

3. Mix the goat cheese, ricotta, ¾ tsp of pepper, basil, 1½ tsp of salt, eggs, and ½ cup of the Parmesan with

an electric mixer and make sure the paddle attachment is on a low speed.

4. In a 9 × 13 × 2-inch baking dish, grease with 1 cup of marinara. Place ⅓ of the vegetables on top. Fit a layer of noodles, a third of the ricotta mixture, a third of the mozzarella into large dollops between the mozzarella. Do it twice but start with the marinara.

5. The remaining 1½ cups of marinara should be spread on top and the last ½ cup of Parmesan should be sprinkled on top as well. Line a sheet pan with parchment paper and put the dish in it. Bake it for 60 to 70 minutes. Let the lasagna become brown and bubbly. Let stand for 10 minutes before serving.

Grilled Mushroom Quesadilla

Total servings: 1

Ingredients to Use

- 1 chopped clove garlic

- 4 ounces of rinsed and sliced mushrooms

- 2 tortillas

- 1 tbsp oil

- 2 tbsp white wine

- ½ small sliced onion

- ½ cup of grated Fontana cheese

- 1 tbsp of parsley

- ½ tsp of thyme

How to Prepare The Meal

1. Use a pan to heat the oil. Put in the onion and mushroom.

2. Sauté the mixture until it is fully caramelized. This may take 20-30 minutes.

3. Mix in the thyme and garlic. Sauté until the fragrance rises for about a minute.

4. Use the broth to deglaze the pan. Make sure it is sautéed until the liquid is absorbed. Bring away from the heat and add the parsley.

5. Melt butter into the pan

6. Swirl the butter around with a tortilla and repeat with another tortilla.

7. Sprinkle some cheese on the tortilla. Add in the onions and mushrooms then top it with the leftover cheese and yet another tortilla.

8. Let the quesadilla cook until it gets golden brown on both sides with melted cheese.

Tip

You can use other melty cheese like mozzarella, Monterrey Jack, Swiss, etc.

North Carolina Sweet Potato Pie

Total Servings: 8-10

Ingredients to Use

- 3 medium-large sweet potatoes
- ½ tsp of salt
- ½ tsp of cinnamon
- Enough pie pastry to make a 9 to 9½ inch deep dish pie shell
- ¼ tsp of ground cloves
- ⅔ cup of packed light brown sugar
- ½ cup of heavy cream
- 1 tbsp of all-purpose flour
- ½ tsp of nutmeg
- ¼ cup of unsalted butter
- ¾ tsp of vanilla extract
- 3 large eggs and 1 egg yolk, at room temperature
- ⅓ cup of granulated sugar
- ½ cup half-and-half or light cream

How to Prepare The Meal

1. Make the pie dough and keep it refrigerated for almost 1½ to 2 hours before you roll it.

2. After that bake the potatoes. Set the oven at 400°F. Line your baking sheet with foil or parchment and put your scrubbed potatoes.

3. Prepare the pie dough and refrigerate it for at least 1 ½ to 2 hours before rolling. Pierce all of them many times using a paring knife. Allow it to bake for 60 to 75 minutes until they become tender. Cut open and let cool.

4. As soon as the potatoes become cool or warm, spoon out the flesh and blend it to form a smooth puree in a food processor. Store 1½ cups of puree in another container keep the rest safe.

5. Flour a sheet of wax paper lightly, then roll the dough on it to form a 13-inch circle. In a 9- or 9 ½-inch deep-dish pie pan, turn the pastry over it. Let it stay in the center, then tear off the paper.

6. Tuck in the pastry properly to fit the pan. Avoid stretching it then make the ridge and flute with the dough that sticks out. Use a fork to poke the bottom of the pie shell for about 6-7 times. Keep in the refrigerator for 30 minutes or 15 minutes in the freezer.

7. Set the oven to 375°F before you start. Get a 16-inches long aluminum foil and use it to fit the pie shell gently so that the dough won't be affected. Make the shell fit the pie like a glove. Lay up the dried beans to a thick layer.

8. Place the pie shell to be baked on the center oven rack. Allow it to bake for 25 minutes. When it is ready, take out the foil and beans with care. If the holes are filled in, poke them again. Replace the shell and bake for extra 6-8 minutes. Take out the pie shell and place it on a cooling rack. When it has cooled, plug the holes with sour cream or cream cheese. Don't discard the beans because you can reuse it.

9. Let the temperature of the oven be at 375°F. The eggs and yolk should be whisked until they become foamy. Mix in the brown sugar, vanilla, sweet potato puree, half and half, sugar, cream, and vanilla. Mix with an electric mixer set at low speed and blend till it is even. Make a mixture of cinnamon, flour, salt, cloves and nutmeg in a small bowl. Blend, after spreading it on the filling and pour it inside the pie shell. Remember to use low speed.

10. After 20 minutes of baking, let the temperature reduce to 350°F and allow it to bake for more than 30 to 40 minutes. To know if it is ready, the pie will feel wobbly and there will be no trace of liquid when you gently touch it. The pie will be more puffy on the sides than the center. Allow it to cool on a rack. Always refrigerate leftovers.

Roasted Cauliflower Soup

Total Servings: 4

Ingredients to Use

- 1 sliced onion
- Salt and pepper
- 4 tbsp of the olive tree extra virgin olive oil
- 1 cup of Farmdale thickened cream
- 1 whole cauliflower (shred into florets)
- 1 tbsp of fresh thyme leaves
- 2 cloves of garlic, crushed
- 1L of Chef's Cupboard Vegetable Stock

How to Prepare The Meal

1. Set the oven at 175°C before using

2. Make a mixture from 2 tbsp of olive oil, the florets, pepper, and salt. Roast in the oven for 10-12 minutes on an oven tray until it is fully caramelized. Stir it at intervals.

3. Use olive oil to sauté the sliced onion in a stockpot. Make sure the onions do not change color.

4. Put in the fresh thyme leaves and remain a little for the garnishing. Cook for 2 minutes more.

5. Put in the vegetable stock. Let it boil for a while before you put in the roasted cauliflower.

6. After it has cooked, let it simmer for 15 and until the cauliflower softens. You can put off the heat and cool slowly.

7. After it cools, return to the stove and add more cream. Let it simmer. You can taste it and check if the seasoning is enough.

8. Serve in bowls and use the cauliflower, cracked pepper, thyme and olive oil that remains to garnish it.

Flavorful Cantaloupe Gazpacho

Total Serving: 1

Ingredients to Use

- 2 cups of cherry tomatoes
- 1 small cucumber, finely diced
- 4 tbsp of olive oil plus extra for drizzling
- 1 ½ pound of peeled, seeded and chopped cantaloupe melon
- 4 slices of prosciutto
- 3 thinly sliced spring onion
- ¼ tsp of red pepper flakes or to taste
- salt, black pepper to taste
- ½ tbsp of apple cider vinegar
- Minced garlic cloves

How To Prepare The Meal

1. Blend the garlic, melons, and tomatoes in a blender until it is very smooth.

2. Mix in the olive oil, apple cider vinegar, and red pepper flakes. Add your seasoning, salt, and black pepper.

3. Blend to mix them. Cover it and put it in the refrigerator until it is served.

4. Place your non-stick frying pan to heat on medium heat. Put in the prosciutto and cook for 1-2 minutes each side until it is crisp.

5. Dish out the gazpacho and use the spring onions, cucumber, and prosciutto as toppings before drizzling with extra olive oil.

Swiss-style Bircher Muesli

Total Servings: 4

Ingredients to Use

- 1 grated green apple,

- 1 tsp of vanilla extract

- 1 cup of whole milk

- 1 juiced lemon

- 2 cups of rolled oats

How to prepare The Meal

1. 1. Mix every single ingredient together and allow it to stand overnight in the refrigerator.

2. 2. The oats will become very hydrated after 12-24 hours. You can then eat them with maple syrup with some little milk or crack.

Basic Vegetable and Chicken Wonton Soup

Total Servings: 8

Ingredients to Use

- 1 tbsp of minced fresh garlic
- ½ cup of finely chopped yellow onion
- ½ cup of sliced green onions
- 2 tbsp of toasted sesame oil
- 1 tbsp of minced seeded jalapeño
- 1 ¼ tsp of kosher salt, divided
- 6 cups of unsalted chicken stock like Swanson
- 7 ounces of shiitake mushrooms
- 4 smashed garlic cloves
- 2 cups of water
- 1 large egg
- 1 cup of diagonally cut sugar snap peas
- 1 cup of diagonally cut carrots
- 1 (1-in.) piece of fresh ginger, sliced
- 32 round of wonton wrappers

- 1 tbsp of minced peeled fresh ginger

- ½ tsp of black pepper

- 12 ounces of ground chicken

- 2 tbsp of rice vinegar

How to Prepare The Meal

1. Turn on a large Dutch oven to medium-high heat. Sauté minced ginger, yellow onion, jalapeno and minced garlic for 4 minutes. Turn in the mixture to a medium-sized bowl.

2. De-stem the mushroom. Slice the mushroom caps thinly and put them differently. Put the black pepper, stems, vinegar, 2 cups of water, stock, smashed garlic, sliced ginger, and 1 tsp of salt into a pan to boil. Cover it and reduce the heat to simmer for 45 minutes. Drain the stock mixture in a bowl and throw the solids out. Put the stock back in a pan that is still on low heat or check instructions for freezing.

3. Put the remaining chicken, ¼ tsp salt, and egg into the onion mixture and stir properly.

4. Use the Wonton wrapper one at a time while making sure the rest are covered to prevent drying. Scoop about 2 tsp of chicken mixture in the middle of the wonton wrapper. Make the edges moist with water, pack up and fold the wrapper edges to form a purse. Keep doing the procedure for the wrappers

and the remaining chicken mixture. You can choose to refrigerate at this point or continue with step 4.

5. Simmer the carrots and the stock in the pan for 4 minutes. Add the dumplings, peas and mushroom caps. Let it cook for 8 minutes. Share the soup into 8 bowls and spray green onions on them.

How to Freeze

Mix the stock and vegetables and allow it to cool completely. Separate the stock mixture and dumplings and freeze them.

Thaw: set the microwave at medium heat, put in the stock mixture for 3 to 4 minutes.

Reheat: turn the stock mixture into a large Dutch oven and simmer for 5 minutes or as long as it takes to heat. Add frozen wontons and allow them to cook for 3 minutes.

Roasted Root Veggies Breakfast Tacos

Total servings: 6

Ingredients to use

- ½ tsp of salt
- 4 parsnips, peeled and cut into ¼-inch (6-mm) dice
- 2 sweet potatoes, peeled and chopped
- 1 tbsp of ground cumin
- 1 tsp of ground coriander

- 2 tbsp of canola oil

- ½ tsp of chili powder

For the lime-cilantro cream:

- ¼ cup (⅓ oz./10 g) of finely chopped fresh cilantro, plus more

- ½ cup (4 oz./125 g) of sour cream

 For the garnish;

- Salt and freshly ground pepper, to taste

- Juice of 1 lime

For the tomatillo salsa:

- 10 to 12 small corn tortillas, warmed

- 6 tomatillos, husked and halved

- ¼ cup (⅓ oz./10 g) of fresh cilantro leaves

- 1 garlic clove

- Salt and freshly ground pepper, to taste

- 1 jalapeño chili, halved lengthwise and seeded

- ¼ white onion, roughly chopped

How to Prepare the meal

1. Set the oven to preheat at 450°F (230°C). Use a parchment paper to coat a baking sheet. In a bowl, add up the parsnips, sweet potatoes, cumin, chili

powder, salt, oil, and coriander. Stir properly to coat the vegetables.

2. Preheat an oven to 450°F (230°C). Line a baking sheet with parchment paper. Pour the mixture into the baking sheet and arrange the vegetables in one layer. Roast it but stir only once. Stop at 20 minutes or when the vegetables are caramelizing.

3. Make the lime-cilantro cream. Mix in the sour cream, lime juice and ¼ cup of cilantro. Stir well and add pepper and salt to taste.

4. For tomatillo salsa, heat up a broiler. Set up the jalapeno and the tomatillos on the baking sheet, cut side down. Broil for about 7 minutes. When it is cool, blend the garlic, cilantro, tomatillos, onion, and cilantro until it is pureed. Add pepper and salt and move it to a smaller bowl.

5. Use the cilantro to decorate the lime-cilantro cream. It's served by placing 3 tbsp of the root vegetables on all of the tortillas one after the other. Dress to top with salsa and serve.

Chicken and Brown Rice Risotto

Total Servings: 6

Ingredients to Use

- 1 cup of chopped cremini mushrooms

- ½ tsp of sea salt

- 6 cups of chicken stock

- 2 tbsp chopped fresh basil

- 2 tbsp of olive oil

- 1 cup of frozen peas, thawed

- ¼ cup of chopped flat-leaf parsley

- 1-½ cups of short- or medium-grain brown rice

- ½ cup of grated Parmesan cheese

- 4 boneless, skinless chicken thighs, cubed

- 2 tbsp of butter

How to Prepare The Meal

1. Warm the chicken over low heat using a medium saucepan

2. Mix 1 tbsp of butter with olive oil and heat in a 3-quart saucepan over medium heat. Put in the mushrooms and chicken thighs and sprinkle Sea salt on it. Cook the mixture and keep stirring until the mushrooms become soft. This can take about 5 to 6 minutes.

3. Put in the rice. Allow it to cook for 4 minutes, stir while cooking. Divide the chicken stock into two and add one part. Continue cooking and stirring until it is soaked for 4 minutes. Change the heat to low.

4. Keep adding the stock in ½-cup portions. Make sure to stir at intervals. Continue adding stock because the rice keeps soaking it up until it becomes tender in 50 - 55 minutes.

5. Add the peas and allow it to cook for about 2 minutes. Put in the Parmesan cheese and the last 1 tbsp of butter. Let it cook for 2-3 minutes so that the butter and cheese are melted.

6. Put in the basil and parsley and stir it. Dish it out immediately.

Breakfast

Banana and blueberry oatmeal

Oatmeal is a great breakfast option for people suffering with acid reflux. Rolled oats are low in fat and sugar and high in protein, making them a perfect grain option to replace white bread or sugary cereals. The fresh fruit adds the perfect balance of sweetness to round out this quick breakfast meal.

Nutritional Information:

Calories: 128 g

Total fat: 4 g

Sodium: 112 mg

Total carbohydrates: 21 g

Fiber: 3 g

Sugar: 4 g

Protein: 4 g

Time:

10 minutes

Serving Size:

½ cup (yields 2 servings)

Ingredients:

½ cup rolled oats

1 cup unsweetened coconut milk

½ banana, sliced

¼ cup blueberries

¼ teaspoon cinnamon

Directions:

1.   Add rolled oats, coconut milk, and cinnamon to a saucepan over medium-high heat. Bring to a boil.

2.   Turn heat to low and simmer to thicken, around four to five minutes. Stir continuously to prevent sticking or burning.

3.   Transfer to a bowl and top with bananas and blueberries.

Apple pie oatmeal

This oatmeal is a healthy take on apple pie you can enjoy for breakfast or even as a late night dessert if the craving strikes. Unlike apple pie, it is low in sugar and fat. Like apple pie, it features warm baked apples and cinnamon, and it's totally delicious. Enjoy this guilt-free taste of an old classic.

Nutritional Information:

Calories: 149 g

Total fat: 5 g

Sodium: 5 g

Total carbohydrates: 28 g

Fiber: 5 g

Sugar: 12 g

Protein: 3 g

Time:

10 minutes

Serving Size:

½ cup (yields 2 servings)

Ingredients:

½ cup rolled oats

½ cup unsweetened coconut milk

1 apple, cored and sliced

1 tablespoon unsweetened applesauce

½ tsp cinnamon

½ teaspoon olive oil

Directions:

1.   To a saucepan over medium heat, add olive oil, sliced apple, and cinnamon. Use just enough olive oil to prevent sticking.

2.   Stir frequently until soft and the outside is golden brown, about five minutes. Remove from pan and set aside.

3.   Turn heat up to medium-high and add in oats and coconut milk. Bring to a boil, then lower heat to a simmer and allow to thicken for four to five minutes.

4.   Stir in cooked apples and applesauce. Transfer to a bowl and serve warm.

Skinny omelet

Egg yolks are high in fat and cholesterol, which takes fried and scrambled eggs off the menu, but it doesn't mean you can't still enjoy a nice omelet.

This recipe uses measurements for the liquid egg whites you can purchase in cartons, which are great to have on hand for acid reflux since egg yolks are usually a trigger food. If you only have whole eggs on hand, the omelet uses about three eggs' worth of egg whites. Be sure to carefully separate the whites from the yolks in a separate bowl or mixing cup before adding them to the pan.

Nutritional Information:

Calories: 241

Total fat: 15 g

Sodium: 223 mg

Total carbohydrates: 13 g

Fiber: 8 g

Sugar: 3 g

Protein: 17 g

Time:

 10 minutes

Serving Size:

1 omelet (yields 1 serving)

Ingredients:

½ cup egg whites

½ avocado, sliced

½ cup button mushrooms, sliced

½ cup baby spinach, chopped

Directions:

1.   Spray a skillet with avocado cooking spray and turn heat to medium-high.

2.   Pour in egg whites. Spread chopped spinach and mushrooms evenly across the top of the egg whites.

3.   Cook for about six to eight minutes. Use the back of your spatula to gently push the edges of the omelet away from the sides of the pan until the eggs stiffen and hold their shape.

4.   Fold the omelet in half and transfer to a plate. Top with sliced avocado.

Bell pepper omelet

Fresh veggies make for a nutritious addition to any breakfast. Make bell peppers the star of the show for an omelet with a bright pop of color. If you prefer slightly firmer peppers, reduce cooking time by a minute or two. Liquid egg whites are used in this recipe to lower the fat content, but if whole eggs are all you have available, the bell pepper omelet can also be made with the whites of three eggs, carefully separated.

Nutritional Information:

Calories: 119

Total fat: 4 g

Sodium: 205 mg

Total carbohydrates: 8 g

Fiber: 2 g

Sugar: 5 g

Protein: 14 g

Time:

 15 minutes

Serving Size:

1 omelet (yields 1 serving)

Ingredients:

½ cup egg whites

¼ cup green bell pepper, diced

¼ cup red bell pepper, diced

½ teaspoon olive oil

Directions:

1. Warm olive oil in a skillet over medium-high heat. Add red and green bell peppers and sauté until tender, about three minutes.

2. Add egg whites to a bowl and stir in mixed bell peppers, mixing until evenly spread throughout egg whites.

3. Return to skillet and cook for six to eight minutes or until eggs are firm. Use the back of a spatula to separate eggs from the sides of the pan while cooking.

4. Fold the omelet in half and transfer to a plate to serve.

Coconut and berry smoothie

This smoothie is perfectly tailored to prevent acid reflux. Packed with anti-reflux ingredients like ginger and aloe vera, this smoothie is as good for your health as it is tasty. Because it uses naturally sweet fruit and coconut water, you don't need to add any refined sugar, which helps to keep symptoms in check.

Nutritional Information:

Calories: 75

Total fat: 2 g

Sodium: 128 mg

Total carbohydrates: 14 g

Fiber: 5 g

Sugar: 8 g

Protein: 2 g

Time:

 5 minutes

Serving Size:

8 ounces (yields 2 servings)

Ingredients:

1 cup coconut water

¼ cup raspberries, frozen or chilled

¼ cup blackberries, frozen or chilled

¼ cup strawberries, frozen or chilled

1 tablespoon aloe vera

1 tablespoon chia seeds

¼ teaspoon ginger, grated

Directions:

1.   Add coconut water, raspberries, blackberries, strawberries, and aloe vera to a blender. Blend for one minute.

2.   Add in chia seeds and ginger. Blend for an additional 20 seconds or until desired consistency is reached.

Watermelon smoothie

Watermelon is a very low acid fruit that is packed with plenty of flavor. It is great for combating acid reflux, and in this smoothie it is paired with other healthy options like spinach and cucumber to keep your morning heartburn-free. Enjoying this sweet smoothie hardly feels like being on a diet at all.

Nutritional Information:

Calories: 92

Total fat: 3 g

Sodium: 7 mg

Total carbohydrates: 14 g

Fiber: 3 g

Sugar: 8 g

Protein: 3 g

Time:

5 minutes

Serving Size:

8 ounces (yields 2 servings)

Ingredients:

1 cup unsweetened almond milk

1 cup watermelon, cubed

½ cucumber, peeled

½ cup baby spinach

1 tablespoon chia seeds

Directions:

1.   Add almond milk, watermelon, cucumber, baby spinach, and chia seeds to a blender. Blend until desired consistency is reached in 30-second intervals, about one minute total.

2.   If desired, chill in the freezer for five minutes before enjoying.

Raspberry breakfast bar

Store bought breakfast bars can be packed with added sugars and acidic ingredients. Ditch the additives and make your own breakfast bars instead, complete with a tangy raspberry jam topping. These bars are good for acid reflux but don't skimp on sweetness by choosing naturally sweet ingredients. These are great to prepare on a slow weekend and enjoy throughout the week, as they make for a wonderful grab and go breakfast.

Nutritional Information:

Calories: 153

Total fat: 6 g

Sodium: 67 mg

Total carbohydrates: 22 g

Fiber: 4 g

Sugar: 6 g

Protein: 4 g

Time:

 25 minutes

Serving Size:

1 bar (yields 6 servings)

Ingredients:

1 cup rolled oats

1 cup cashews

1 cup raspberries

1 cup pitted dates

1 tablespoon chia seeds

1 teaspoon vanilla extract

½ teaspoon honey

½ teaspoon pink Himalayan sea salt

Directions:

1.   Begin by preparing the raspberry jam topping. Add raspberries, chia seeds, and honey to a food processor. Pulse until smooth, around 30 seconds, and transfer the jam to a bowl.

2.   Allow the jam to sit for about 15 minutes so it can thicken.

Meanwhile, begin preparing the bars, starting by rinsing the food processor and wiping it dry with a paper towel.

3.   Add oats to the food processor and process for about one minute.

Add cashews, vanilla extract, and sea salt. Process for another two minutes, slowly adding dates one at a time until all ingredients are incorporated.

4.   In a baking pan or stiff-sided storage container, press about ¾ of the mixture uniformly into the bottom, packing well. Spread the raspberry jam evenly over the mixture and top by crumbling what remains of the mixture.

5. Cover and refrigerate to store, and let the bars chill for at least one hour before cutting for best results.

French toast

White bread contains added sugars that can agitate acid reflux symptoms, which means it is restricted in an anti-reflux diet. However, this doesn't mean bread is entirely out of the question. This French toast recipe uses whole grain bread and easily digestible ingredients like lowfat yogurt and coconut milk. You can use liquid egg whites for this recipe, or you can use the whites of two eggs, carefully separated. On a lazy weekend, this is the perfect decadent breakfast to start the day off.

Nutritional Information:

Calories: 135

Total fat: 2 g

Sodium: 200 mg

Total carbohydrates: 22 g

Fiber: 3 g

Sugar: 7 g

Protein: 8 g

Time:

 25 minutes

Serving Size:

2 slices (yields 2 servings)

Ingredients:

2 thick slices of whole grain bread, cut diagonally

⅓

cup unsweetened coconut milk

¼ cup egg whites

¼ cup lowfat yogurt

¼ banana, sliced

1 teaspoon vanilla extract

½ teaspoon cinnamon

Directions:

1.   Add coconut milk, egg whites, vanilla extract, and cinnamon to a wide bowl and whisk until well combined.

2.   Heat a skillet over medium heat.

3.   Dip the slices of bread into the egg mixture and liberally coat each side. Transfer bread to the skillet.

4.   Cook about four minutes on each side so that French toast turns golden brown. Let cool on a plate and top with yogurt and sliced bananas.

Snacks and desserts

Spinach and artichoke dip

Store bought and restaurant spinach and artichoke dips are usually high in fat, but you can make your own using whole ingredients and low fat alternatives. Spinach and artichoke dip is a creamy, savory snack that can be made in larger batches and eaten in portions throughout the week. Keep in mind that this recipe uses a small amount of low-fat cheese, so be cautious if cheese is a trigger food for you. Enjoy this dip with whole grain crackers, chunks of sourdough bread, a small vegetable assortment, or simply eat by the forkful if you are so inclined.

Nutritional Information:

Calories: 77

Total fat: 5 g

Sodium: 176 mg

Total carbohydrates: 4 g

Fiber: 2 g

Sugar: <1 g

Protein: 4 g

Time:

 35 minutes

Serving Size:

⅓ cup (yields 8 servings)

Ingredients:

2 cups unsweetened coconut milk

2 cups artichoke hearts, chopped

1 ½ cups baby spinach, chopped

½ cup low fat parmesan cheese, shredded

1 tablespoon olive oil

Directions:

1.	Preheat oven to 350 degrees Fahrenheit.

2.	In a saucepan, combine olive oil and coconut milk. Over medium-high heat, bring to a boil and then reduce heat to medium-low.

Simmer for about three minutes, just until thickened.

3.	Stir in parmesan cheese and mix well to melt. Add artichoke hearts and baby spinach. Heat for another two minutes.

4.	Transfer to an oven-safe baking dish. Bake for about 30 minutes or until top is bubbly, and allow to cool before serving.

Carrot fries

French fries are filled with unhealthy fats as a result of the deep frying process, not to mention the added sugar when dipped in ketchup, but you can beat fry cravings with these healthier carrot fries. You can make them right in your oven, no other tools needed and with minimal prep work.

Carrot fries work great as a side for another dish or as a snack on their own.

Nutritional Information:

Calories: 42

Total fat: 3 g

Sodium: 493 mg

Total carbohydrates: 4 g

Fiber: 2 g

Sugar: 1 g

Protein: <1 g

Time:

35 minutes

Serving Size:

24 fries (yields 5 servings)

Ingredients:

1 pound carrots

1 tablespoon olive oil

1 ½ teaspoons pink Himalayan sea salt

1 teaspoon ground black pepper

1 teaspoon ginger, grated

1 teaspoon rosemary

1 teaspoon parsley

Directions:

1.   Preheat oven to 425 degrees Fahrenheit.

2.   Wash and peel carrots. Cut into strips about ¼-inch thick, around the same size as a standard French fry.

3.   Add olive oil, sea salt, pepper, ginger, rosemary, and parsley to a bowl and mix. Toss carrots in the mixture until well coated.

4.   Line a baking sheet with aluminum foil. Spread coated carrots out across its surface and drizzle the remaining oil mixture overtop.

5.   Bake for about 30 minutes until carrots are tender but not overly soft and mushy.

Crackers and almond butter

Sometimes simple and easy is the best way to go. These crackers are extremely easy to prepare in no time at all, but they're still packed with flavor. The almond butter is filling, so even a few crackers is enough to hold you over until your next meal. Feel free to customize these with other acid reflux-friendly fruit toppings like blackberries or pears.

Nutritional Information:

Calories: 237

Total fat: 13 g

Sodium: 114 mg

Total carbohydrates: 15 g

Fiber: 5 g

Sugar: 5 g

Protein: 7 g

Time:

 5 minutes

Serving Size:

4 crackers (yields 1 serving)

Ingredients:

4 saltine or soda crackers

2 tablespoons almond butter

¼ apple

¼ banana

Directions:

1.	Wash and core apple. Divide into slices, and cut slices in half. Slice the banana into four even-sized pieces.

2.   Spread about ½ tablespoon of almond butter on each cracker. Top with chopped apple and sliced banana and enjoy.

Watermelon sorbet

Watermelon is great for acid reflux and it packs plenty of sweetness. Store-bought ice creams and sorbets contain tons of sugar, but watermelon is so naturally sweet and tasty that this recipe requires no added sugar at all.

When choosing a watermelon, pick one that feels weighty in your hands.

Also, look for melons with a pronounced yellow spot known as a field spot, which is where the melon rests on the ground when growing. Ripe melons will have darker yellow, almost orange, field spots; these will provide the sweetest pieces of watermelon.

Nutritional Information:

Calories: 67

Total fat: <1 g

Sodium: 3 mg

Total carbohydrates: 16 g

Fiber: 1 g

Sugar: 13 g

Protein: 1 g

Time:

 10 minutes/overnight

Serving Size:

1 cup (yields 4 servings)

Ingredients:

3 cups watermelon, cubed and chilled

1 cup water

¼ cup unsweetened coconut milk

Directions:

1.   Add cubed watermelon to a blender. Pulse until uniform, about 30 seconds.

2.   Pour in water and coconut milk and blend to combine for another 30 seconds.

3.   Transfer to a freezer-safe dish and chill overnight. Scoop into balls with an ice cream scoop or large spoon to serve.

Coconut pudding

This coconut pudding recipe combines the delicious taste of coconut with fresh raspberries for a tasty treat. Coconut is great for reducing heartburn symptoms and keeping acid reflux in check, so it is a good choice in any dessert. You can also top this pudding with your choice of reflux-friendly fruits.

Nutritional Information:

Calories: 60

Total fat: 4 g

Sodium: 16 mg

Total carbohydrates: 8 g

Fiber: <1 g

Sugar: 4 g

Protein: 2 g

Time:

 15 minutes

Serving Size:

½ cup (yields 6 servings)

Ingredients:

3 cups unsweetened coconut milk

¼ cup raspberries

1 tablespoon coconut flakes

2 teaspoons gelatin

1 teaspoon honey

1 teaspoon vanilla extract

Directions:

1.   Pour coconut milk into a saucepan and heat on medium-high. Stir frequently and bring to a boil.

2.   Reduce heat to low to simmer. Stir in gelatin and allow to thicken for 10 minutes, continually stirring.

3.   Remove from heat and mix in honey and vanilla extract. Allow to cool before transferring into serving bowls or refrigerator-safe containers if chilling is desired. Top with raspberries and coconut flakes when served.

Peach pops

Fresh peaches are sweet and tangy, which makes them perfect as a dessert component. You can also use frozen peaches for this recipe, but fresh ones will pack slightly more punch in terms of flavor. While they are slightly acidic, peaches are still relatively low in acid, so they should be able to be enjoyed on an acid reflux diet. Though unlikely, pay attention to any possible symptoms after eating these pops to know if peaches are a trigger food for you.

Nutritional Information:

Calories: 33

Total fat: 1 g

Sodium: 76 mg

Total carbohydrates: 8 g

Fiber: <1 g

Sugar: 7 g

Protein: 3 g

Time: 30 minutes/overnight

Serving Size:

1 ice pop (yields 6 servings)

Ingredients:

1 cup peaches, chilled or frozen and thawed

⅔ cup nonfat yogurt

⅓ cup lowfat cottage cheese

1 teaspoon honey

Directions:

1.   Puree peaches in a blender for about 30 seconds.

2.   Add yogurt, cottage cheese, and honey to blender and blend for another 30 seconds, until the puree is uniform.

3.   Pour into popsicle molds or dixie cups and freeze overnight for best results.

Lunch and dinner

Tuna salad pita

Sandwiches aren't out of the question on an acid reflux diet as long as you are smart about what you put on them and what type of bread you use.

Ingredients like tuna and wheat-based breads like pita are informed choices you can make to keep heartburn at bay during lunchtime. This recipe swaps out mayonnaise for nonfat yogurt to make the tuna salad, as the vinegar and lemon juice components of mayonnaise can aggravate acid reflux symptoms.

Nutritional Information:

Calories: 266

Total fat: 1 g

Sodium: 287 mg

Total carbohydrates: 21 g

Fiber: 2 g

Sugar: 4 g

Protein: 40 g

Time:

 10 minutes

Serving Size:

½ sandwich (yields 2 servings)

Ingredients:

1 pita bread, halved lengthwise

1 cup tuna

½ cup nonfat yogurt

½ cup spinach

1 tablespoon dijon mustard

Directions:

1.   In a bowl, combine tuna with nonfat yogurt and dijon mustard.

2.   Spread tuna mixture over one half of the pita bread and top with spinach. Close sandwich and cut into halves.

Chicken soup

Chicken soup is the perfect warm lunch for a chilly afternoon or a sudden illness. It's great to prepare over the weekend and enjoy throughout the week. If you have leftover baked chicken from another meal, save time by repurposing it for use in this recipe. Be careful to choose a chicken broth that does not contain high amounts of garlic and onion as these can cause acid reflux symptoms.

Nutritional Information:

Calories: 288

Total fat: 13 g

Sodium: 502 mg

Total carbohydrates: 16 g

Fiber: 6 g

Sugar: 2 g

Protein: 29 g

Time:

 50 minutes

Serving Size:

1 cup (yields 6 servings)

Ingredients:

4 cups low sodium chicken broth

1 pound boneless skinless chicken thighs, diced

1 15 ounce can black beans

3 celery stalks, sliced

3 carrots, sliced

4 tablespoons ginger, grated

Directions:

1.   Add diced chicken thighs to a skillet over medium heat and cook until brown, about 10 minutes. Stir frequently to prevent sticking and burning.

2.   Transfer cooked chicken to a large stockpot and pour in chicken broth. Bring to a boil on high heat, then reduce heat to low and simmer for 15 minutes.

3.   Drain black beans and add to the broth, alongside celery, carrots, and ginger. Cook for about 20

minutes to soften vegetables and infuse flavor into the broth, stirring occasionally. Ladle the soup into a bowl and serve hot.

Beef stew

Beef stew is best served as a weekend dish with leftovers used as lunch throughout the week due to its slightly longer cooking time. Absent of typical heartburn triggers in beef broth like tomatoes and onions, this recipe is a tasty and hearty meal that is good for you too. Onion substitutes like leeks or shallots can be added if tolerated, but be sure to test whether or not these ingredients give you acid reflux symptoms before adding them.

Nutritional Information:

Calories: 201

Total fat: 6 g

Sodium: 1021 mg

Total carbohydrates: 26 g

Fiber: 4 g

Sugar: 2 g

Protein: 13 g

Time:

 1 hour

Serving Size:

1 cup (yields 6 servings)

Ingredients:

2 cups water

1 pound carrots, peeled and sliced

½ pound lean flank steak

½ pound red potatoes, peeled and cubed

½ cup button mushrooms, diced

¼ cup whole wheat flour

½ tablespoon soy sauce

2 teaspoons pink Himalayan sea salt

1 teaspoon ground black pepper

Directions:

1.   Cut flank steak into cubes. Place in a bowl with flour, salt and pepper and coat well with the flour mixture.

2.   Grease a skillet with cooking spray over medium heat. Add steak cubes to the skillet in small batches to prevent overcrowding and too much liquid building up in the pan. Brown on each side, about five minutes per batch.

3.   Transfer browned steak to a large stock pot alongside water, soy sauce, carrots, and potatoes.

4.   Cook over medium heat until carrots and potatoes are tender and meat is cooked through, about 40 minutes. Stir occasionally to prevent sticking and disperse flavor into the broth. Ladle stew into a bowl and enjoy hot.

Macaroni salad

Pasta made from whole wheat is easier on an acid reflux afflicted stomach than its white flour, refined grain counterpart. With this flavorful macaroni salad recipe, you will hardly taste the difference between the two. If desired, you can switch the sour cream out with nonfat greek yogurt for a similar taste.

Nutritional Information:

Calories: 101

Total fat: <1 g

Sodium: 158 mg

Total carbohydrates: 21 g

Fiber: 3 g

Sugar: <1 g

Protein: 4 g

Time:

 15 minutes

Serving Size:

½ cup (yields 12 servings)

Ingredients:

1 box whole wheat elbow macaroni, about 3 cups uncooked

½ cup fat free sour cream

¼ cup celery, finely diced

¼ cup red bell pepper, finely diced

3 tablespoons parsley, finely chopped

1 tablespoon dijon mustard

1 teaspoon pink Himalayan sea salt

1 teaspoon ground black pepper

Directions:

1.   In a pot over high heat, bring salted water to boil. Cook elbow macaroni according to package instructions, about eight minutes.

Drain the pasta after cooking and rinse until it is room temperature.

2.   In a bowl, mix together sour cream, parsley, dijon mustard, sea salt, and pepper. Stir into pasta.

3.   Mix in celery and red bell pepper. Combine well so that all ingredients are evenly distributed. For best results, chill before eating.

Chicken salad

Chicken salad is incredibly versatile. You can eat it as is, or you can make yourself a sandwich on whole grain bread. You can even use it as the protein for a salad made with fresh spinach and kale. Whatever your preference, this chicken salad recipe made with poached and shredded chicken is easily adaptable for almost any use. You can also cut the chicken into small cubes rather than shredding if desired.

Nutritional Information:

Calories: 85

Total fat: 3 g

Sodium: 153 mg

Total carbohydrates: 2 g

Fiber: <1 g

Sugar: <1 g

Protein: 13 g

Time:

 35 minutes

Serving Size:

½ cup (yields 6 servings)

Ingredients:

1 pound boneless, skinless chicken breasts

½ cup low sodium chicken broth

½ cup celery, diced

2 tablespoons low fat mayonnaise

1 tablespoon rosemary

1 tablespoon parsley

¼ teaspoon pink Himalayan sea salt

¼ teaspoon ground black pepper

Directions:

1. Begin by poaching the chicken. Place chicken breasts in a pan and add chicken broth, rosemary, and parsley. The chicken broth should cover the chicken about halfway.

2. Bring the broth to a boil over medium-high heat. Reduce heat to low and simmer for five minutes.

3. Cover the pan and turn off the heat. Allow the chicken to sit for fifteen minutes.

4. Transfer chicken to a cutting board. When cooled, use two forks to shred the chicken and move to a mixing bowl.

5. Add in celery, mayonnaise, sea salt, and pepper. Fold in the mixture until chicken is coated evenly. Chill in the fridge for about 15 minutes before serving.

Mango chicken salad

Mango is a non-acidic fruit that actually functions as a natural antacid for your body. Take advantage of its unique, beneficial properties with this mango chicken salad recipe, which is the perfect colorful interruption on a busy day. This recipe uses fresh mango, but you can also use frozen mango that has been thoroughly defrosted. Mangos give this salad a natural sweetness, so no salad dressing is necessary.

Nutritional Information:

Calories: 171

Total fat: 3 g

Sodium: 282 mg

Total carbohydrates: 16 g

Fiber: 3 g

Sugar: 12 g

Protein: 21 g

Time:

 30 minutes

Serving Size:

1 cup (yields 4 servings)

Ingredients:

1 pound boneless, skinless chicken breasts

1 mango, diced

1 cup kale, chopped

½ cup low sodium chicken broth

½ cup red bell pepper, diced

1 tablespoon parsley

1 tablespoon soy sauce

1 tablespoon ginger, grated

½ tablespoon thyme

Directions:

1.   Start by poaching the chicken. Add chicken breasts to a pan alongside chicken broth, parsley, and thyme. The chicken broth should cover the chicken breasts about halfway.

2.   Bring to a boil over medium-high heat, then reduce heat to low and allow the broth to simmer for five minutes.

3.   Cover and turn off heat, allowing chicken to sit for 15 minutes. When it is done, move to a cutting board and cut chicken into ¼-inch thick cubes.

4.   In a large bowl, toss kale with diced mango, red bell pepper, and cubed chicken. In a smaller bowl, mix soy sauce and ginger, then drizzle overtop the salad and serve.

Baked chicken nuggets

Chicken nuggets aren't just for kids, especially not when they're prepared in a way that cuts out saturated fats while still remaining delicious. Baking chicken nuggets instead of frying them reduces the fat content, keeping them from irritating your stomach and causing heartburn. A riced cauliflower breading helps to keep refined carbs low, so you can eat these chicken nuggets guilt-free.

Nutritional Information:

Calories: 94

Total fat: 2 g

Sodium: 338 mg

Total carbohydrates: 6 g

Fiber: <1 g

Sugar: <1 g

Protein: 12 g

Time:

 30 minutes

Serving Size:

 5 nuggets (yields 4 servings)

Ingredients:

1 pound boneless, skinless chicken breasts

1 egg

1 cup riced cauliflower

½ cup brown rice bread crumbs

½ teaspoon salt

½ teaspoon ground black pepper

Directions:

1.   Preheat oven to 350 degrees Fahrenheit.

2.   Cut chicken breasts into cubes. Each chicken breast should yield about eight to ten pieces.

3.   Set out two wide bowls. In one, beat the egg and add salt and pepper.

In the other, combine brown rice bread crumbs with riced cauliflower.

4.   Line a baking sheet with aluminum foil or parchment paper. Dip cubed chicken first into the bread crumb mix, then into the egg mix, and then back in the bread crumbs before transferring to the baking sheet.

5.   Bake for 10 minutes, flip chicken nuggets, and bake for another 10 minutes.

Quinoa stuffed chicken

Stuffed chicken is a great vehicle for getting your protein, grains, and veggies all in one bite. This recipe uses lemon zest, but in most cases this should not aggravate your acid reflux. While lemon juice is acidic like other citrus fruits, lemon zest made from grating the rind of a lemon lacks the potent acidity that takes lemon juice off the menu. Used in small amounts, you can enjoy lemon flavor without any of the acid reflux.

Nutritional Information:

Calories: 176

Total fat: 5 g

Sodium: 171 mg

Total carbohydrates: 16 g

Fiber: 3 g

Sugar: 1 g

Protein: 15 g

Time:

 50 minutes

Serving Size:

½ chicken breast (yields 4 servings)

Ingredients:

1 pound boneless, skinless chicken breasts

½ cup spinach, chopped

½ cup quinoa

4 asparagus spears, chopped and stalk ends discarded

½ carrot, sliced

½ lemon

2 ounces feta cheese, crumbled

Directions:

1.   Preheat oven to 350 degrees Fahrenheit.

2.   Rinse quinoa thoroughly, drain and add to a saucepan with 1 cup water. Bring to a boil on medium high heat, then cover and lower heat to a simmer. Cook for 15 minutes, turn off heat, and let sit for five minutes, still covered.

3.   While quinoa is cooking, grease a baking sheet with cooking spray and lay out chicken breasts.

4.   In a bowl, combine spinach, asparagus, carrots, and feta cheese. Use a grater to zest the lemon. Spoon half of the filling mixture onto the middle of the chicken breasts, staying away from the edges.

5.   Roll chicken into a spiral shape and keep closed by inserting a toothpick through each end. Put chicken in the oven and bake for 20 minutes. Be sure to check that no pink remains inside the chicken before serving.

Chicken kabobs

Featuring healthy grilled chicken and acid reflux fighting vegetables, these chicken kabobs are a great dinner option whether you're firing up the grill on a summer evening or in the middle of winter. Kabobs are a great tool for portion control, as not only do they slow down how fast you eat, they also naturally portion out your food.

Nutritional Information:

Calories: 197

Total fat: 7 g

Sodium: 60 mg

Total carbohydrates: 9 g

Fiber: 2 g

Sugar: 7 g

Protein: 25 g

Time:

 35 minutes

Serving Size:

 1 skewer (yields 4 servings)

Ingredients:

1 ½ pounds boneless, skinless chicken breasts

2 cups zucchini, sliced and ends discarded

1 cup button mushrooms, halved

1 cup watermelon, cubed

1 tablespoon olive oil

½ teaspoon parsley, finely chopped

½ teaspoon rosemary, finely chopped

½ teaspoon ground black pepper

Directions:

1. Prior to starting this recipe, soak wooden skewers in warm water for

10 minutes to keep them from burning on the grill. You can also use reusable metal skewers, which require no soaking.

2. Cut chicken breasts into cubes about 1 inch thick.

3. Combine olive oil, parsley, rosemary, and black pepper in a bowl.

Coat cubed chicken in the olive oil mix, and use remaining oil for the mushrooms and zucchini.

4. Thread chicken, zucchini, mushrooms, and watermelon onto skewers, alternating the order as you go and keeping skewers relatively even.

5. Turn grill to medium heat and grill skewers about five minutes on each side or until chicken is cooked through.

Chicken parmesan

Love chicken parmesan, but hate the way the tomato sauce and spices give you heartburn? You can actually make chicken parmesan totally sauceless and still have plenty of flavor in the dish. This recipe uses brown rice bread crumbs, but you can use regular plain or seasoned bread crumbs if they do not agitate your acid reflux.

Nutritional Information:

Calories: 251

Total fat: 6 g

Sodium: 368 mg

Total carbohydrates: 5 g

Fiber: <1 g

Sugar: <1 g

Protein: 40 g

Time:

 55 minutes

Serving Size:

 1 chicken breast (yields 4 servings)

Ingredients:

2 ½ pounds boneless, skinless chicken breasts

½ cup brown rice bread crumbs

1 egg

3 tablespoons low fat parmesan cheese, grated

½ teaspoon pink Himalayan sea salt

Directions:

1.   Preheat oven to 375 degrees Fahrenheit.

2.   Set out two bowls. In one, crack and beat the egg. In the other, combine brown rice bread crumbs with parmesan cheese and sea salt.

3.   Spray a baking sheet with cooking spray.

4.   Dip chicken breasts in egg and then in the bread crumb mixture. Lay chicken out on the baking sheet.

5.   Put in the oven and bake for 40-45 minutes. Check to ensure there is no pink remaining in the chicken before serving.

Turkey burger with mushrooms

Turkey burgers are much leaner than their beef patty counterparts, reducing the harmful fats that can exacerbate acid reflux symptoms. While standard cheeseburgers may be out of the picture, this turkey burger makes for a solid replacement. Don't be turned away by the commonly held misconception that turkey burgers are dry and tasteless; the burger is far from dry, and the simple addition of mushrooms and soy sauce gives the meal powerful flavor that rivals any hamburger.

Nutritional Information:

Calories: 161

Total fat: 11 g

Sodium: 304 mg

Total carbohydrates: 7 g

Fiber: 1 g

Sugar: 1 g

Protein: 9 g

Time:

 20 minutes

Serving Size:

 1 burger (yields 4 servings)

Ingredients:

½ pound lean ground turkey

½ cup button mushrooms, sliced

1 whole wheat hamburger bun

1 tablespoon soy sauce

1 ½ tablespoon olive oil

Directions:

1.   Mix ground turkey with soy sauce and 1 tablespoon olive oil. Shape into four patties, each about ½ inch thick.

2.   On the grill, cook the turkey burgers over medium heat, about five minutes for each side. You can also use a stovetop griddle.

3.   While the turkey burger patties are cooking, heat a skillet over medium heat and add in sliced mushrooms and remaining ½ tablespoon olive oil. Sauté until warm and soft, about three minutes.

4.   Remove burgers from the grill and plate on whole wheat buns. Top with sautéed mushrooms and enjoy.

www.ingramcontent.com/pod-product-compliance
Lightning Source LLC
Chambersburg PA
CBHW060323030426
42336CB00011B/1183